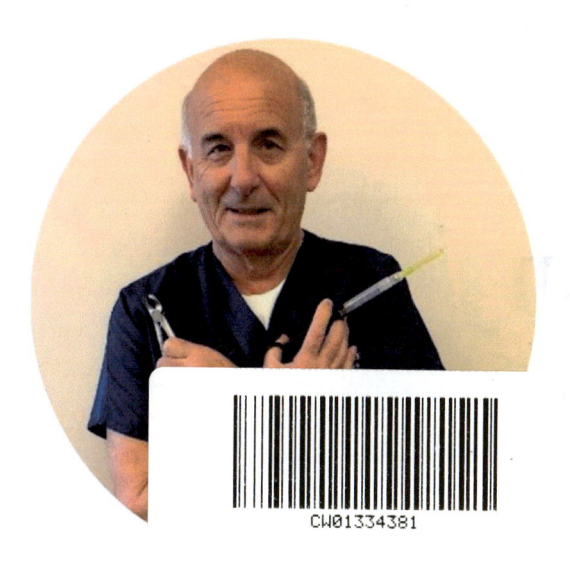

In my early teens, I knew I wanted to become a dentist. Working in the NHS and the private sector, I enjoyed all aspects of a unique profession. My wife, Sue, has been tremendously supportive in this project, together with my three children. I found that fishing on my local river for trout and salmon helped me through difficult times, a hobby that continues to this day. Growing vegetables and teaching karate, as a fifth dan black belt instructor, have also provided valuable relaxation. As I approach retirement, I can look back at some wonderful memories that are worth sharing, recalling the people I have met along my chosen path. All that has enriched my life.

Open Wide was published in 2021.

This is a work of fiction. Names, characters, businesses, places, events and incidents are either the product of the author's imagination or used in a fictitious manner. Any resemblance to actual persons, living or dead, or actual events is purely coincidental.

OPEN WIDER

Dr Bernard Lester
BDS (U.MANC) MJDF RCS

OPEN WIDER

Pegasus

PEGASUS PAPERBACK

© Copyright 2023
Dr Bernard Lester

The right of Dr Bernard Lester to be identified as author of this work has been asserted by him in accordance with the Copyright, Designs and Patents Act 1988

All Rights Reserved

No reproduction, copy or transmission of this publication may be made without written permission.
No paragraph of this publication may be reproduced, copied or transmitted save with the written permission of the publisher, or in accordance with the provisions of the Copyright Act 1956 (as amended).

Any person who does any unauthorised act in relation to this publication may be liable to criminal prosecution and civil claims for damage.

A CIP catalogue record for this title is available from the British Library

ISBN 978 1 91090 393 3

Pegasus is an imprint of
Pegasus Elliot MacKenzie Publishers Ltd.
www.pegasuspublishers.com

First Published in 2023

Pegasus
Sheraton House Castle Park
Cambridge CB3 0AX England

Printed & Bound in Great Britain

For my dear brother Phil who passed away in 2021. He always had a joke to tell and his storytelling was legendary.

I am indebted to all the patients who had stories to share, and to all my staff who helped me remember them, Sue, Pip, Bev and Jean.

To my dearest wife, Sue, who devoted many hours correcting my English.

To Pegasus Publishers, who encouraged me all the way.

Contents

INTRODUCTION 11
UP DOWN AND UP 15
HIGH NOON 30
A LOVE STORY 40
THE LONG SLEEP 54
A LITTLE BOY'S TALE 62
SEXUAL HEALING? 74
BOOK 2 THE NURSES' TALES 87
PIP'S STORY: THE ACCI-DENTAL SAMARITANS 88
BEV'S STORY: THE ACCI-DENTAL DELIVERY? 96
JEAN'S STORY: THE FLYING FIFTY PENCE 100
A VIEW FROM BOTH SIDES OF THE PROBE 104
BOOK 3 111
THE ACCI-DENTAL SLEUTH (IF THE CAP FITS!) ... 112
MY BOOK OF LIFE 123
11. MY TOP TWENTY REQUESTS 127

INTRODUCTION

These stories are loosely based on cases I have seen. I have added some technical detail so that the reader will more understand the issues involved. It is important to note how dentists in general can help and change people's lives for the better.

It is not just about filling teeth. The more severe the damage, especially in bad accident cases, the more challenging dentistry becomes. There can be emotional and psychological issues to deal with, as well as the physical repercussions.

However, in my experience, the dental work carried out can be the final piece in the recovery of any patient, not only restoring appearance, but giving them the confidence to face life again

It has given me and my team immense satisfaction to see patients leave the surgery with a smile, and with normal function of their teeth.

For every patient seen there is always a team at work, be they receptionists, nurses, dentists and technicians. A team that pulls together, as I have always tried to encourage, will give the patients confidence.

This in turn will put them more at ease, help us to get to know them, and produce the best possible results.

Also, from a patient's view, it is important that their contact at the surgery should be a welcoming friendly face, preferably someone they recognise from their previous visit. It is vitally important that dentists rid themselves of the cold sterile atmosphere that often pervaded surgeries in past days. We have all observed this, where the turnover of staff is such that it can make patients uneasy, wondering what can be wrong to cause it. Often patients may not see the same clinician which can cause further anxiety.

Allaying these fears has always been my aim. Trying to understand the people who worked for me, their problems, personal or professional, was always a priority. Regular staff meetings ensured that issues were aired, where patient care was always discussed as the main topic. In this way we were well prepared for most scenarios. I have been immensely fortunate in that I have been blessed with staff who have, in the main, stayed with me for most of my professional life. We have, in effect, all grown up together. Because of this, the surgeries have matured into ultra-professional clinical environments, yes, but with a friendliness and insight into our patients' needs and expectations. This can often be forgotten in today's high-tech and pressured times, where finances are stretched, together with constant litigation fears. The corporate surgeries have a lot to offer, but in my opinion, the lessons I have learned over many years have to be addressed.

Sometimes work did not always go to plan. Crowns did not fit properly or were constructed in the wrong shade. Matching colours was always a fine art which involved all of us checking. If we were not happy, the laboratory remade them. The more complex the treatment, the more each stage had to be as near perfect as possible. If we were not completely happy, we would go back and start again.

Perfection may never be attained, but the most important issue was always how much difference the completed work made to the individual. It may not have been possible to correct every nuance, but if this was explained to the patient, it helped them understand that their expectations sometimes had to be curtailed. We always tried to ensure that they understood any limitations of treatment, and this ensured any rapport began on fertile ground. 'The customer is always right' cannot be applied to dentistry. We spend almost five years becoming qualified clinicians, a fact that is often forgotten, so it is vitally important that all options and costs for treatment are explained. In this way patients can make informed decisions, based on the points discussed. What is possible and what is not should always be made clear, in a concise and intelligible way to avoid misunderstandings. Dentists have had to develop clear comprehension of patient fears and concerns, and alter their manner and behaviour to allay them.

A holistic approach has always been my mantra. I spent time with the patients I saw, just talking about, well anything at first. This way I was able to get to know them, what motivated people to come and see me, above all remembering that they may be really frightened of treatment. It's not hypnotherapy, not rocket science, just old-fashioned common sense — relaxing them, even sharing a joke. Now it's a completely different scenario. I always accompanied them out of the surgery and ensured that all was well. Sometimes in more complex cases I would contact them later to see how they were. Result? Patients stayed with me and remembered always any kindness and empathy shown to them.

However, I can think of very few patients who were disappointed with our dentistry. Thank you cards, small gifts, smiles and sometimes tears said it all.

UP DOWN AND UP

Hans Christian Andersen once wrote "Life is like a beautiful melody, only the lyrics are messed up". I think we can all empathise with these words, but read on and see what you think.

James was a long-standing patient, and I last saw him two years ago, when he was thirty-five years old but looked much older, dishevelled, gaunt and troubled. He put this down to personal problems and so I didn't intrude with any intimate questions. He was however very distressed with the appearance of his now neglected upper front teeth. After a full assessment, I recommended four crowns and two veneers, but the cost was prohibitive and despite our best efforts, we could not arrange for this on the NHS. This is a not an uncommon problem, showing the limits of the system and restrictions dentists are often fighting. He worked as an IT specialist in a well-known local firm of computer consultants, where his wife worked as the personal assistant to the manager.

Now look at him! Immaculately dressed and a golden suntan that smacks of exotic winter holidays. He was bursting with vitality, completely different, except of course for his teeth.

"I've been to hell and back over the last two years and as I regard you as a friend and confidant, I will tell you the whole story but you won't believe it," he said smiling. "Suffice to say I can now afford the treatment you suggested." He continued talking as if he found it a cathartic experience, a release, a cure. "As you know I am into computers, working for Galaxy IT, a company doing really well now!"

My nurse Bev and I certainly wanted to sit down with a coffee and listen to him, but he was booked in for a long appointment! Let me tell you a little about his treatment. Crowns are really a last resort treatment on already heavily restored teeth, and involve two stages. Firstly, we take an impression of both the upper and lower arches, then prepare the teeth and shape them so they are able to accommodate the restorations. This is done with high-speed instruments and the remaining shape should converge slightly towards the incisal edge of the tooth.

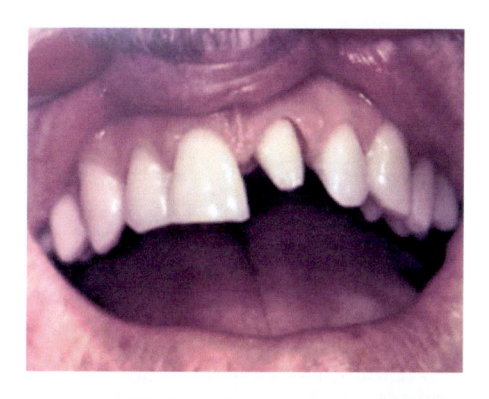

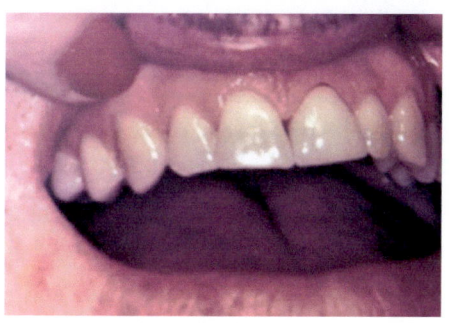

A crown before and after!

We then take a final impression or scan of the finished preparations, check the shade needed and put on temporary crowns. The second stage is a week later where we remove the temporaries, put on the completed crowns and show the patient before final cementation. The veneers are different, needing only minimal removal of the surfaces of the teeth, and these can be done at the same time. Veneers consist of a very thin piece of porcelain or composite, used to alter shades, shape or cover up imperfections. "I'm going to put some local anaesthetic into the area, then we can continue with the treatment," I told James. With a numbing mouth and signs of emotional memories James continued his tale whilst the anaesthetic was taking effect.

JAMES'S STORY:
I was doing really well at work, bringing in new contracts. Promotions seemed certain, and my wife Pamela was kept busy with her PA duties for the boss, Richard Tranter. Idyllic you may think. She was wild when I first met her, but after six months she moved in with me, and we seemed to be happy together. Marriage seemed to be the most natural thing in the world to us, and so with all our friends and family present, we tied the knot. That was six years ago. We had even been talking about moving to a bigger house and starting a family. On a weekend before Christmas, Richard went to a conference in Manchester and insisted on taking his PA, my wife, with him. I thought nothing of this at the time, and after a couple of days she returned home after what she described as an "intensive weekend". From this time on I noticed significant changes in her behaviour which on hindsight should have been a warning. It was our wedding anniversary but Pamela was at another IT meeting with her boss about fifty miles away, and so she decided to stay over for the night. "We can celebrate another time. I simply have to go," was her parting comment. The eternity ring,

exquisite in design with diamonds around a central sapphire was my present, to remain in its box awaiting her return. Maybe not, I thought, I'll drive down and surprise her, maybe stay for dinner then drive home, or stay with her. Excitedly, I prepared my overnight bag, and drove on expectantly into the night.

"I'm going to start the crowns now," I explained to James. The impressions had been taken; we were ready to go. I removed the old fillings and replaced them with a special cement. The teeth were shaped and tidied; we were ready for the final stages. The special silicone impression of the preparations was taken and the temporary crowns made by using the mould of the original teeth before we started, but hey, we wanted to hear more of the story, so a short break!

James continued by telling us about his emotions on the trip to the hotel where his wife was staying.

"I felt really excited at the thought of surprising Pamela, maybe a romantic evening and more. It had been a long time since we had been away together, any intimacy was rare, something I tried to ignore — putting it down to our high intensity jobs. As the journey continued and I neared my destination, I started to feel uneasy, a strange sensation in the nerves deep inside me, not butterflies, more a sense of apprehension. No, this was only the excitement at seeing her and presenting the ring. Yet there was a trepidation, strangely like the feeling I'd had on the day I married. Those happy memories flooded into me, drowning the negative vibes that had been there a moment before, and I drove into the hotel car park like a teenager on a first date, excited, nervous and full of a strange anxiety.

It was eight p.m. as I walked into the busy reception as people were flooding into the hotel. Should I surprise her at the bar? Yes, try that first, I thought. It was crowded and I entered unnoticed, looked all around the dimly lit area but could not see Pamela, so I considered trying the restaurant. As I walked out something in one of the alcoves caught my eye, something that looked familiar, a black leather jacket with gold buckles. I stopped and peered into the alcove. Disbelief, shock, I felt my skin burning and my heart pounding. There in the corner Pamela and Richard, together in a passionate embrace, his hands furtively exploring her thighs, whist she pulled at his hair. I stepped back, tried to come to terms with what I saw and walked outside, breathing heavily and in a trance like condition. Had I really seen them together? I took out my phone and dialled Pamela's number.

"Hello darling," she answered after some time. "Are you okay, is anything wrong?"

In my best unemotional voice, I blurted out a reply. "Just phoned to see how you are."

"I'm exhausted. Had a hell of a day so going straight to bed. Are you sure you're okay, you sound odd."

"Yes, I'm fine, I'll see you tomorrow night." My legs were still trembling and my heart thumping as I watched them from a discreet distance walk hand in hand, oblivious to anybody around, through to the bedrooms. I slowly followed, protected by a constant stream of staff and guests. Then they stopped at one room. Would they go in together or was this a flirtation only? No, they entered together. I stood transfixed not knowing what to do for a length of time lost to me. I walked up to their door and waited in the now deserted corridor. I listened to two people in what I can only imagine was a conjugal embrace,. The sound of them losing themselves in each other pierced me to the depths of my soul, a memory which has stayed with me, though no longer haunts me as it did at that moment. I knocked on the door, the noises stopped. "Who is it?" Richard inquired. I didn't answer but knocked again. I could hear footsteps, then the door opened. Without thinking I pushed into the room. There was Pamela half naked with her hand to her mouth and face contorted.

"Oh no," she gasped. I glared at them both. They could see the fury in my face combined with an emotion I do not want to feel again. "Happy anniversary!" I muttered and threw the ring at her.

I turned to face a subdued Richard, fists clenched, rage in my eyes. I stared at him. "You will find that sometimes the wanting is better than the having." The next thing I remember was driving home with constant calls from Pamela, and messages I never read, such was my distress. I threw the phone into the first bin I came across.

I collected a few things I needed from home, left the car and walked. All feelings and emotions had been wrenched from my soul, leaving a barren landscape, incapable of rational thought. All I wanted to do was disappear from my life as it was, hoping maybe that some sort of normality would eventually return.

"I'm ready to fit the temporary crowns now," I explained, but it was as if James was back in that dark time in his life and could not break free from it. "That's fine, we'll just give it a few minutes to set." The purpose of temporary crowns is to act as a cover to protect the teeth and usually gives a good appearance whilst the finished crowns are fabricated.

James continued, "I walked all over the country for six months until I realised that I had run out of any form of cash or credit. Now it's difficult to explain what it feels like to be homeless, sleeping on the street, or trying to find a place to wash or use a toilet. It can be frightening as desperation takes over. Picking discarded food from bins, hoping that people would give you a little cash for a hot drink. This was my lowest point. My only release came when I would fall into that dark sea of oblivion, called sleep. When you are at rock bottom there are plenty of bumps and you realise that you cannot sink any lower, there is only one way to go."

I explained to James we were finished for this appointment and he was to return to have his crowns fitted the following week. Bev and I felt as if we had been reading a good book, a real page turner that made us wonder how this story was going to end.

James returned a week later, my last appointment of the day, usually reserved for more extensive work where we were not restricted to time. He was wearing a designer suit and looked at ease with life. "Okay, James, I am going to put some local anaesthetic in place so there should be no discomfort when we remove the temporary restoration." Taking off these provisional plastic type crowns is not always straight forward, and sometimes they need to be divided to remove them. The remaining teeth can also be quite sensitive. "All right, James, if you like please continue with the story whilst the anaesthetic takes fully." James could not wait to resume and continued where he left off as if there had been no interruption.

"It was a freezing cold morning; my legs were stiff and getting up from the pavement and my blankets was difficult. "Hello," said a gentle voice. "I've bought you a hot coffee." There were two people standing in front of me, a woman about my age, slim, dark hair with a disarming smile, and a man perhaps a little older, well over six feet tall, heavily built and hands like shovels. "My name is Abby and this is my brother Tom." We walked and talked for the rest of the morning, Abby explained that they too had decided to leave the world behind for reasons I never found out until much later. Abby said they had seen me on the street several times and wondered if they could help, a sort of camaraderie found with rough sleepers. They bought me food and took me to a homeless shelter where strangely I found some rare stability.

"You need a job," Abby said. I found an intriguing beauty in the gentle, genuine and undemanding way she talked to me. Tom, a contented giant of a man, always backed her up with, "I agree". The two of them reminded me of characters from a Charles Dickens novel. I washed and spruced up, and caught sight of myself in the mirror, a little shoddy with my now slender frame and non-designer stubble. The last months had taken their toll. Abby took me to a residential home for the elderly and introduced me to the manageress who she seemed to know very well. "He needs a job. He's clean, intelligent and hardworking, I will vouch for him." The manageress Jane, a stout woman with a round, smooth friendly face, asked me about my experience in care. "Just my mother before she died, four years ago." Whatever was discussed prior to my visit seemed to impress Jane and I was given my duties, night-care mainly. Over the next few weeks, I was trained in the care for those frail people and some became good friends, one resident especially. Her name was Helen Parr, a charming elderly person full of life. Abby and Tom came every few days to visit me and gradually I was becoming more human. "Remember," Abby said smiling, "fate is the cards that you are dealt in life, but destiny is how you play them".

"Okay, I'm just taking off the temporary crowns, then we'll try everything in." When they were all in place retained by what we call a try in paste, I showed James." Wow! Please fit them permanently," was all he said. Firstly, I fitted the veneers, a delicate process which involves lightly etching the surface of the teeth with a very dilute acid and then bonding them in place with a special cement cured by an ultra violet light. We then fixed in the crowns and I removed any excess. "I want to give you twenty minutes to get used to them and see if you have any problems. Why don't you continue with your story?" Bev smiled.

I became very attached to Helen especially when she regaled me with tales from her childhood, her two husbands she outlived, and her son from her first marriage, who she did not want to talk about. I never asked why because there was an obvious distaste and change in her demeanour when discussed, indeed she never even mentioned his name. Helen was having trouble sleeping one night and so we sat and chatted. For the first time I opened up about my troubles and why I found myself in this situation, fifty miles from where I left my life. Strangely, Helen listened intently and asked me about Richard and paid particular attention to the business details and name. I took this to be no more than an old lady wishing to show the same concerns for me as I did for her, which was immensely satisfying.

We continued for three months with a now well-established routine. I would spend time talking to the residents and finding out about their experiences, lives, loves and fears. Helen seemed in really good spirits and said there was something she needed to discuss when I had time. I saw Abby and Tom on my days off, joining them as they toured the areas where there were rough sleepers. It was at this time that Tom pulled me to one side and explained the abuse that they had endured as children, and how they had been forced to leave their home and wander the streets. He had told Abby that he would never leave her side until he was sure she was safe from any further abuse. One evening in July, I returned for my shift at the care home to be met by Jane weeping uncontrollably. "Helen has died. One moment she was here having tea, then she was gone". Helen had been like a second mother to me and I felt the same feelings of grief and loss. Her last instructions were that she was to be cremated with nobody present.

It was as if life had put the brakes on again, I felt myself drifting backwards. Two weeks later I received a letter from Helen's solicitor and executor of her will, asking me to attend his offices, which I duly did.

He read the will. "I leave all of my estate, the sum of £50,000 to James who has cared for me in a way which I never thought I would experience. I also leave him my business Galaxy IT, presently run by my son from my first marriage, Richard Percival Tranter". The poor solicitor thought I was going to faint, and offered me some tea. I needed something stronger. I apologised and said I was just shocked and couldn't come to terms with all the unbelievable issues involved. There was a struggle with all my emotions, as if it was a battle to see which one came out on top, with me helpless to control the situation. Finally, the solicitor put aside his professional air, searched a drawer, and found a bottle of so-called medicinal brandy. "To be used for emergencies!" he joked.

I was stunned and it took me some time to come to terms with my new situation. I had a meeting with Abby and Tom and explained all to these two wonderful Samaritans. "I have a plan," I said. Abby smiled and held my hand. This was the first time our relationship had taken on any form of intimacy, and led to a closeness and reciprocated love I thought I would never find again. Tom was really pleased for us both. "Now about this plan…" he said, his confidence and strength filling me with an inner determination. In this life of snakes and ladders, it was as if a giant spiritual hand had propelled me upward away from all my troubles.

The day arrived. I let Helen's solicitor organise the meeting, and apparently Richard had been informed of his mother's death plus the fact he was not mentioned in Helen's will. I can only imagine, gleefully, what he was now thinking.

The staff, some twenty or so had been informed of the meeting and to expect the new owner to be in attendance. I was standing in a hidden part of the room where I couldn't be seen but I had a clear view of the scene, and there was Pamela looking gaunt and strained standing next to Richard fidgeting nervously in anticipation. I thought then that the relationship was under pressure. This was the moment, nearly two years after that awful night, here I was. The wheel had certainly come full circle! "I want to introduce you all to your new owner," the solicitor said quietly. "He will explain the changes that will be made." I stepped forward. There were gasps from the staff, many of whom I knew well. Richard and Pamela were transfixed, pale, shocked, speechless, mouths open, staring at me as if I was some sort of apparition, which I suppose I was.

Tom appeared at my side. "As you know my name is James, and I am going to leave the running of the business to my new manager Tom. He will tell you all about the staff changes," I said with a transfixed glare at my ex-wife and her partner. The room was silent. Pamela and Richard left and I watched them through the window arguing vehemently outside. I wanted to store the events of the day so that I could open them up at any time to remind me of life's strange twists. Revenge yes but no satisfaction in watching them, more a sadness that sometimes life can be like a bottle thrown into the ocean, tossed around by the waves.

Bev and I were spellbound! "Thank you for sharing the tale. It was some story!" I walked James to the reception where he was met by an adoring woman who complimented him on his new smile.

"Thank you, Bernard, I'm delighted with my new teeth and feel complete again. Can I introduce you to Abby, my soon to be fiancée?"

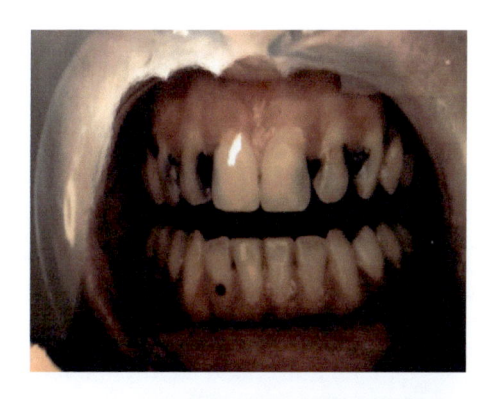

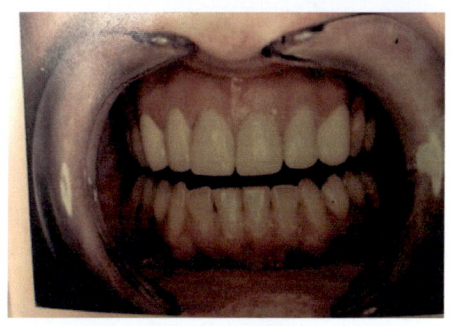

**HELLO AND GOODBYE JAMES,
NOT BAD EH?**

HIGH NOON

So, you think old people in care homes are just biding time in 'God's waiting room'? Not so! I have met some of the most astute and complete people over many years in these residences. However, time takes its toll on us all, and occasionally stories are told to you that make you just sit up, take notice and admire the tenacity and bravery of the older generation.

Margaret was a lovely vivacious lady in her mid-eighties. Agile mentally, but not too good physically. I saw her regularly to keep her denture in good condition, but it was becoming obvious that major treatment was going to be needed, and completed at my surgery. She had a group of three very close friends who always sat by whenever I attended her.

When I last saw her at the care home, I explained that I had done everything possible to keep her denture and remaining teeth in reasonable condition but explained that decisions had to be made about the way forward. However, on this occasion, she looked frailer than I remember, had bruises on her arm and had "misplaced" her false teeth. This immediately flagged up a warning of possible abuse. Margaret knew exactly what I suspected but insisted that all was well, and she would return to the surgery as soon as possible to have the recommended treatment completed. Strangely she said that she and her friends, had a job to complete first, then winked at me.

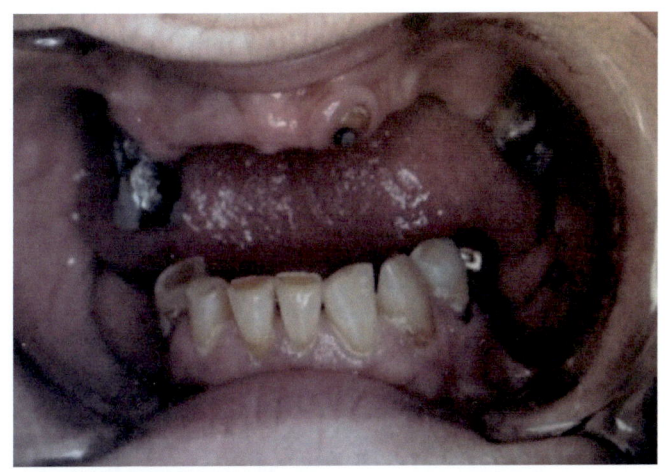

MARGARET PRE-TREATMENT

Margaret came into the surgery to discuss her treatment plan. There was a big change in her demeanour. Gone was the bruising, she looked more at ease and physically well. She had no upper denture and all her remaining teeth were heavily restored, or severely damaged. Her lower teeth now needed urgent attention. The joint decision was made to complete a full denture on the upper jaw and to save as many teeth as possible on the lower. Over eight visits we completed the work for her and she was delighted with the result, but gradually over the period the story of her trauma had unfolded.

A little about her treatment first. Making a denture involves up to six appointments starting with impressions then making wax blocks to determine the height of the teeth and register the correct biting position. Only then can teeth be added, tried in and completed. The extractions are done at the same time as the final visit.

In the case of Margaret, we then completed several crowns on the severely damaged lower teeth. Is it worth it on a person of this age you may ask? Actually, yes. It is important to listen to the patient, no matter what age, suggest the options for treatment and then discuss them fully before a decision can be made. The treatment that Margaret had received made a significant difference, not only to her appearance, but to her quality of life.

Over these appointments Margaret apologised if she gave the impression that she was ignoring my advice, and explained why in a kind of serial.

MARGARET'S STORY:
Jacob Valance was the manager of our residential home. He was overweight, had alcohol-fumed bad breath and a body odour that defied belief. In other words, he did not have a lot going for him. However, he was clever, a bully and he was known for "borrowing" food from the kitchen. Of late some of the residents had complained of money disappearing from their rooms. Complaints to

the staff went unheeded and we never saw the owner. Worst of all, he occasionally roughly handled the residents, which is why my arm was bruised. Bernard, I could not mention it then but suffice to say it's been sorted.

I have three very close friends at our home, and we shared meals and tales from our past. Recently they were becoming more subdued because of Jacob's dictatorial behaviour. Cecil, Clint and Barbara were the closest I had for family, and so it was natural I would want to protect them.

Cecil had been a car thief for most of his life, or as he preferred to be called, "a specialist car mechanic". A slight man in stature, with thinning grey hair contrasting with intensely blue eyes. He was clever and loyal to his friends but suffered from occasional debilitating Tourette's syndrome which caused him to have repeated bouts of swearing. I think that was the reason he had been shunned by his family. A heart of gold did not come close to describing this gentle man.

Clint was of West Indian origin. He was larger than life, had been tall but now stooped and a chemical engineer before his retirement. He always said that the thing he enjoyed most was converting beer, wine and Scotch into urine. He insisted on doing this every day. His real name was Clive but he was fascinated by old Western cowboy films, strolling around the home like Clint Eastwood with a hat to prove it, hence his nickname "Clint".

Then there was Barbara. An ex-woman police constable, well known and loved in the area, but now afflicted with an anxiety that was debilitating, preventing her from community life, except with her three friends. She was loving and affectionate, with an occasional glint in her eye that suggested an interesting life. Clint was besotted with her and we had lost count of how many times he had proposed marriage.

It was a Sunday morning. We were sitting at the breakfast table waiting for Cecil who was a little late. Then we saw and heard him coming towards us. "Fluck, fluck, my flucking dentures have gone flucking mithing again and I can't flucking speak properly, let alone eat anything, fluck!" He didn't realise it but this wonderful human being was soon going to be our hero.

Over the next week the situation became worse. Our false teeth were constantly mixed up, then went missing, much to Jacob's amusement. Then they just disappeared. This coincided with more food finding its way to his car as we watched the daily thefts. The abuse continued as well as my bruising, the laughter and mocking of Cecil, the money thefts. Something had to be done. Barbara ruled out the police because it would be difficult to prove, and so it was left to the four of us to become the architects of his downfall.

It was up to me to utilise all our individual skills to bring Jacob down, and so I devised a scene in my head that was feasible for us. So the 'Four Horsemen of the Apocalypse' went to work.

The day came, the plan was put into action and each of us had a part to play. Jacob usually left work at six p.m. and so we carefully organised our day. Firstly, Cecil our 'car mechanic' had to break into Jacob's car and what he did will come to light later. Suffice it to say that after twenty minutes when the manager was out of sight, he returned to us. "Well?" I said. "How did it go?" "No flucking problems. All flucking done. The boot is just slightly flucking open, plus a few flucking tricks I've learnt from my old flucking trade." Somehow Cecil sounded so lovable without his teeth!

Barbara had been filling small plastic coin bags with icing sugar and sealing them. Twenty should be enough she thought. As Jacob always took two bottles of water from the fridge before he left, it was her job to make sure that there were only two there at that time. She was careful not to be seen and so I distracted some of the now curious residents. She had to half fill the bottles with a combination of a laxative, no, more a purgative that Clint had made up from his past knowledge. "Routine," he said. "But he will only have ten minutes before dire effects." It was an unfortunate choice of words. Now the main event. He had to fill the car boot with various items, wallets plus a Lladro ornament from my room, whist making sure the boot had enough 'stolen' items in it. Most importantly, he had to put the sugar sachets in a prominent position, not too obvious, but seen if searched. Barbara watched Clint move off his chair when Jacob was not to be seen.

"Clint," she said," if you pull this off I'll marry you!" He was ecstatic, put a small cigar in his mouth and sang "Do not forsake me oh my darling, on this our wedding day." Mild applause from the residents who were old enough to remember *High Noon* with Gary Cooper.

It was thirty minutes later I saw Clint coming back just as Jacob barged into him pushing him to one side. I actually thought he was going to hit poor Clint, but no he got out of the way humming the theme from the *Good, Bad, and the Ugly,* whilst still keeping his cigar and hat in place. Perfect, just like Clint Eastwood, I thought.

Barbara had one more job to do, but that would be saved until just before Jacob left, and so we waited. At 5.40 p.m. Jacob came out of his office in a foul mood, again pushing everyone out of the way and swearing constantly. His eyes were bloodshot and I was sure he had been drinking. Bang on cue, he went to the fridge and picked out the last remaining water bottles. "You," he shouted at one of the staff, "fill the fridge with more water." I sighed in relief, then chuckled as he downed a whole bottle of 'water'. Clint who was now mentally arranging his wedding to Barbara, saw this and gasped. "He's got fifteen minutes maximum."

Barbara made her call to the local police station where she was well known, explaining the situation that he may well have been drinking, and we were 'concerned!'

"Cecil," I asked, "tell me exactly what you did to the car, apart from opening the boot and removing a back light."

Cecil looked indignant. "I cannot flucking giph away the tricks of my flucking trade, but okay, I filled the windscreen washer bottle with flucking beer, adjusted the electrics so it will squirt the beer out at an angle whenever he flucking turns off the flucking engine, or flucking starts it." This lisp he had gave him such a wonderful persona!

The last we saw of Jacob was when we heard a screech of wheels as he accelerated away from the drive just in front of our home. Now the wait!

The police arrived about two hours later to speak to Barbara and explain exactly what had happened. They insisted on speaking alone with her, but with a mischievous smile she explained that her friends would want to hear what happened and stay.

We sat around the police officer, Clint nuzzling up to Barbara, and Cecil doing his best not to interrupt the proceedings with various expletives.

The officer continued, saying that after a 'tip off' from a concerned member of the public, they stopped the said vehicle, and asked the driver to turn off the engine and step out of the car. As he did this the windscreen washers squirted what appeared to be alcohol of some kind into the face of his sergeant. At this point they were becoming concerned with the aggressive manner of the driver, plus the pervading smell of alcohol. They were then asked by the driver, who seemed to be in some physical discomfort and holding his stomach, why he had been stopped. They explained that a back light was missing on his vehicle. At this point they asked the driver to sit in the back of the police car. His sergeant then opened the boot of his car, finding various items and wallets with names of people, apparently from this residence. Of more concern were several small sachets of what appeared to be drugs for distribution. These were taken for analysis. There were large amounts of packaged food in the boot with the name of this home on them. After eventually contacting the owner, they found that he did not have permission to remove these items. Further, after a breath test, he was found to be over the limit, which was not a surprise as there was a constant smell of beer in the car.

As they continued to question him, he suddenly yelled with pain and this was accompanied by a strange gurgling explosive noise. At this point he and his sergeant left the car to get some air! This most disrespectful action was the last straw. They arrested him for being in charge of a vehicle whilst under the influence of alcohol, theft, driving an unsafe vehicle, and finally soiling the seat of a police car. According to the owners, he would not be returning as manager.

Barbara thanked her son, the attending officer.

It was time for some drinks to celebrate. I filled all the glasses and proposed a toast. "To Cecil." Without his expertise this would not have been possible. To

Clint, our cowboy who will always be known as "The man who 'shopped Jacob' Valance of his liberty" to quote John Wayne? And to Barbara, never underestimate her.

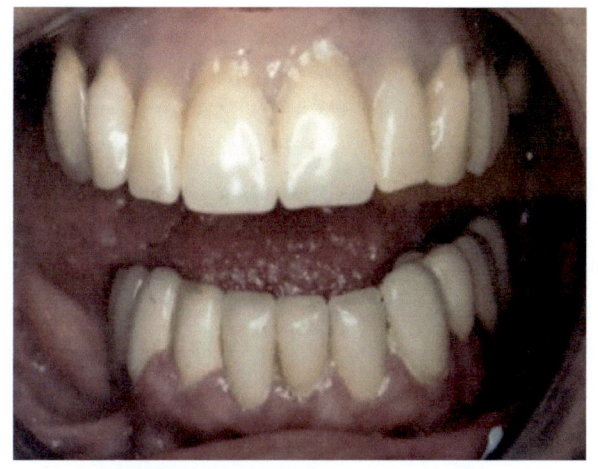

MARGARET, POST VALANCE

A LOVE STORY

Serge Lippmann was a new patient, born in 1918 in France, making him 82 years old when I saw him. He had a wonderful French lilt added to his Mancunian accent, as well as a round strong face full of character and adventure, and a body that showed a good level of fitness and care. He must have been well over six feet tall, with no tell-tale stooping or lack of mobility. However, he had neglected his teeth over the years but most were still present and his bone structure belied his age.

He wanted to improve the appearance of his teeth and did not want a denture. He did not tell me why he suddenly decided to overcome his dental phobia, but said it would become apparent after the treatment. Now in a case like this, the general support of the teeth and condition of the gums has to be ascertained first, and if any disease of the gums (gingivitis), or supporting bone (periodontitis) is present, this has to be dealt with before any restorative care.

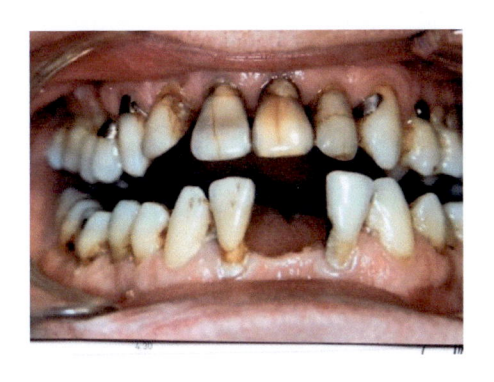

SERGE PRE-TREATMENT

Strangely, Serge had a tattoo of SS on his right forearm which seemed at odds with his Jewish background. He noticed me staring at it with horror but then he gently placed his giant hand on mine and said, "I will explain as we continue with the treatment."

After we had stabilised his gingivitis with specialised hygienist consultations, thus ensuring that the remaining teeth were ready for conservation, we settled on a treatment plan that involved crowns on his upper teeth, extractions of the two lower incisors next to the gap, then the provision, after healing, of a lower six-unit fixed bridge. This involves crowns on the two supporting teeth at either side of the space, with dummy teeth attached to replace those extracted and previously lost. I asked him how he lost his lower front teeth, and he smiled and looked at me as if to say "you will not believe it." I never got an answer until much later in his story. There were three sections of treatment. Firstly, we would extract the two lower incisors with a nil prognosis, that means beyond conservation, then complete the crowns on the uppers. After the lower jaw had healed, I would complete the bridge to fill the gap.

"I want to tell you how I lost the two lower teeth," Serge said. "But I must tell you the full story." I am sure I detected tears in his eyes when he said this. Bev, my nurse, also seemed aware of his emotional memory.

We popped a local anaesthetic into the lower tissue around the two teeth to be extracted, an articaine-based drug, very effective. Serge then started, without being asked, his story of such power and effect that it both saddened and also filled us with hope at the same time.

SERGE'S STORY:
I lived in Reims, France, the son of a baker and patisserie maker, Lippmann's, together with my older sister and younger brother. It was hard work and as the days rolled by, I could see that I would have to move on in order to supplement the family income. I searched for places that needed a good baker, but in France this was becoming difficult. By chance I heard that there was a shortage in Germany and so I managed to contact a friend of my father, Chaim Aischberg, who had a shop in Cologne. I spoke good German and I thought this would be an adventure. Chaim was a lovely man and so in February 1938 I arrived at his shop in a mixed area of Cologne. He made me very welcome and allowed me to stay in the flat above the shop, so I was never late for

work! His bagels were special, and people from all over the area and all religions would gladly queue for them.

He treated me very well but I detected a fear in him whenever black booted soldiers walked past the shop glaring in. "There is going to be trouble, I can sense it," he would say.

In May, 1938, I went home to Reims to see my family. At my father's shop one morning, I saw her. A young woman who I knew I was fated to meet, and according to my sister her name was Michel Rose Bloch. She was slim and her long hair wisped about her face, with wonderful eyes that made me shiver. She had a voice that was full of confidence and a smile that said we belonged together. Suffice to say we hit it off immediately, became close friends, then even closer. We married in October and she decided to return with me to Germany where we lived for a cosy few weeks in our flat above the shop. Chaim made us very welcome, but he looked even more anxious than I remember.

"Serge I am just going to extract the two teeth now," which I duly did. He remained seated whist we checked that he was comfortable with full haemostasis (bleeding stopped).

On his next appointment which was scheduled for two hours, he looked calm and with an easy smile he said, "Will it be okay to call you Bernard? I will feel easier."

"You can call me anything you want to Serge."

We started on the upper crowns. The teeth were very heavily filled and decayed so not only did I have to shape the teeth, but all the old fillings and any recurrent decay had to be removed, then to be replaced with dressings. After the usual surface and local anaesthetic, impressions and shade taking, I began the preparations. Then Serge continued.

It was November seventh 1938, when a Polish Jewish student was accused of shooting a German diplomat, Vom Rath in Paris. It made all the headlines. Little did we know that two days later, the infamous Kristallnacht would occur. On the night of November ninth, 1938, we were just closing the shop when all the front glass was shattered, with shouts of "Juden".

We were terrified when we looked out and saw a crowd yelling and screaming, whilst the police looked on, even seeming to encourage the mob. Then came the worst feeling of all as a fire was started inside the shop. Within minutes it engulfed the old wooden structure and we had no time to collect any belongings. We dashed out into the street and what happened next is burnt into my memory.

As Rose, Chaim and myself escaped through the front door, two soldiers rushed forward. One hit Rose with the butt of his rifle, knocking her to the ground. It was a melee with the rabble drunk on hatred. I could not reach my poor wife, but Chaim did his best to help her as I turned to face the soldier as he laughed. He was much smaller than me and I could see the sudden fear in his eyes as I grabbed him by the throat. I squeezed hard until I saw the life drain out of him as his eyes bulged. I can only now imagine his thoughts at being killed by a Jew. Was this murder? No, this was war! And only the beginning. I turned and struggled to find Rose, but the next thing I remember was being hit hard and losing consciousness.

I awoke after two days in a house I didn't recognise, with lower teeth missing and blood streaming from my head. Chaim was there tending to me as best he could. "Rose, I said, where's my little angel?"

Chaim with tears in his eyes told me what happened. "It was the mob that separated her from us and I saw her taken and forced into a truck filled with Jewish neighbours. I only managed to escape because the fire spread panic, and in this vision of hell all I could do was pull you away as the crowd surged forward, their faces contorted in a weird dance of hate. I could not save her; I am so sorry my dear friend. All I know is that if we go back, we will be arrested and interned in what they call a concentration camp."

What I later found out was on that night about thirty-thousand German Jewish citizens had been taken and incarcerated.

We returned to the shop in darkness to find it deserted and burnt out. Chaim found two of his neighbours who had been hiding nearby and warned them to leave immediately because the dead German soldier had been found. The SS were now combing the area. They had already taken prisoners and shot them in retaliation. One was a young woman who fitted the description of Rose together with a young boy.

I was distraught and Chaim pulled me away as in a fit of grief and fury I went to find her body. "If you go anywhere near the police, you will be shot. We must return to France."

These were indeed words of wisdom. As we manoeuvred our way through the narrow streets there was a movement ahead. "Halt oder ich schiebe!" (Halt or I will shoot.) As we ran a single bullet shot rang out and my friend dropped beside me. As Chaim died his final words were "Go and live a good life. Don't hate. Remember if you want revenge dig two graves." Then he was gone.

All the preparations were complete, impressions taken and temporary crowns fitted. A subdued Serge left to return in one week. I looked at my nurse Bev, and said, "This is some story!"

Serge returned in good spirits and so I explained that the next stage would be to remove the temporary crowns and fit the final restorations. During the procedure, he continued his story.

I left my friend where he died, as something in me said that my life had to go on. I travelled at night and after many days I arrived home. Our families were distraught and heartbroken with my news, and I realised I could not stay. I was determined to help my country in whatever way I could. I joined the army and soon settled into a different life. I trained to be with special forces and was made a sergeant. On the day I was promoted my squad insisted on tattooing my arm SS... Sergeant Serge!

War broke out and on the twenty-first of June 1940, France surrendered. After this it was not a good time to be a Jew in the French army. I was unable to contact my parents and felt uneasy about them, but my commanding officer told me not to go to try to find them, and instead secretly flew myself and ten colleagues to England.

The English army appreciated my skills and we joined a French commando group. We were sent all over occupied France and Belgium, and later in the war to Germany. On one occasion I was only a few miles away from my home in Reims, but no, I was under orders. This was a bloody part of my life that I do not want to talk about or try to remember. Bernard, you fortunately have never been in a war, fighting for freedom to preserve your way of life. I cannot explain what it is really like, the destruction, the shootings, watching some of my colleagues and friends die as we sabotaged many parts of the German war effort. All I can say is that when I look around at the democratic values that we cherish in this country, it was worthwhile.

I fitted the crowns and showed him. "That's wonderful, almost a gentleman," he said. After he left the surgery, I asked Bev if she had any idea how this story would end. "Very sadly or possibly not," was her guarded reply.

It was now time to construct the bridge to fill in the gap in Serge's lower arch. This involves crowning the teeth on either side of the gap, then constructing six porcelain bonded to gold crowns, joined together in one piece. In this way the two crowned teeth act as supports. As ever Serge arrived on time and we started with the usual anaesthetic, impressions for the temporary crowns, together with matching shades for the teeth. Serge continued with his story, but both Bev and I were so far unable to unravel this intriguing tale.

It was the thirteenth of April 1945 and we were in Germany outside the town of Celle. Together with other SAS units we were to liberate Belsen, a notorious prison camp. Our job was to watch the camp from a distance and not interfere until the British SAS had entered, followed by the army. Even at a distance I thought it was a bad dream, with the horrors I saw as I watched through binoculars, unable to intervene.

One particular guard caught my attention, a tall woman who seemed to tower above the poor souls she was in charge of, smiling as she threatened a woman and two children with a pistol. Then three shots rang out. I could not believe the act of sheer brutality that I had just witnessed and I found myself weeping uncontrollably as I thought that this had been my Rose's fate, so long ago now. That terrible empty sadness was replaced with anger.

British forces liberated Bergen-Belsen on the fifteenth of April 1945. Thousands of bodies lay unburied around the camp and some sixty thousand starving and mortally ill people were packed together without food, water or basic sanitation. Many were suffering from typhus, dysentery and starvation. Nearly fourteen-thousand prisoners would die after liberation. Some seventy-thousand had already perished at this camp, including 15-year-old Anne Frank, a month before the SAS arrived.

I entered the camp with my colleagues and saw just what the Nazis were capable of first hand. There was a truce around the camp area, but fighting was still going on beyond this. I could not stop thinking about my wife and just hoped that she had not suffered any of the inhumane treatment I witnessed.

As I wandered around the camp, I saw a group of now disarmed Germans, and yes, there was the tall female guard, arrogantly strutting around, as if she was just "doing her job".

"Wo sind die Leichen der Mutter un der Kinder, die du erschossen hast? (Where are the bodies of the mother and children you shot?) She was astonished that I spoke fluent German, and replied saying all bodies were taken to a special grave, or left. "Heil Hitler" was her parting comment with a click of her heels. That was the only time I lost control as I dragged her to a pit full of rotting corpses, put my pistol to her head and said, "Dies ist ein Jude den du nicht toten wirst. Du verdienst es nicht zu leben!" (This is one Jew that you will not kill. You do not deserve to live.) As I threatened her with the gun pointed at her head, I saw the fear in her eyes, and wondered how many people she had killed who felt that same unbelievable, unfathomable terror. I wrapped my finger around the trigger determined to seek some retribution, but then a thin emaciated hand gently moved the gun away. It was a man, a prisoner, tattooed number on his arm, just skin and bone. Our eyes locked together and in that few seconds I truly realised the horrors that he had endured. I lowered the gun and turned around as a group of both men and women survivors pounced on the guard. I didn't look back but I do know that her body was not buried with any of the dead inmates of this hell on earth, out of respect to them.

We had finished the treatment and once again Serge was full of emotion, as were we, but said he would be okay and return in a week to have the treatment completed.

The final bridge for Serge was ready, and we carefully removed his temporary crowns and then placed the final restoration in position to show him. "I am so pleased; I cannot remember when I last had teeth of my own." All the checks were done and we were ready to complete the cementation. I chose the correct luting material and held his new teeth in place until fully set. After tidying up, Serge wanted to finish his story.

Typhus was a killer in the camp and the makeshift hospitals were full of distressing cases. The doctors had lists of names of those too ill to be moved and it was my job to try to find out what nationality they were. You have no idea how many there were. I separated them as best I could.

I came to the French list and looked at all the names, possibly a family I knew. Suddenly I noticed a Michael Bloch and wondered if he was related to my dearest Rose. It was only when I realised that this patient was in the women's section that I felt my whole body tremble. My heart pounded and my mouth went dry. Michael? Or Michel? No, it couldn't be! It was just a clerical error. It would have said Lippmann on the list, and so convinced myself that I was wishing for a miracle.

The doctor in charge asked me if anything was wrong. "No, I'm fine," I said and asked him where this patient was. I walked along the row of makeshift beds, with doctors and nurses doing their best to keep these poor souls alive. Many were barely recognisable because of their diseases and malnutrition. As I passed rows upon rows of the atrocities the Nazis had perpetrated, I found myself once again straining to prevent myself taking further retribution in some way. I kept control as I realised what I had already had to do to make it this far. Yet as I walked past the endless patients I was overcome with a primeval emotion deep within.

Then I stopped. In the makeshift bed in front of me was a woman, pale, emaciated and with eyes that said she was near the end. I looked at the name on her records. "Michael Rose Bloch, or Lippmann." I sank to my knees and held her hand. She turned towards me, with nothing in her eyes, then suddenly a tear, recognition and a smile. Her hand stretched weakly to meet my face. Was I too late? "Rose," I pleaded. "You have survived this far, don't let go now please." She was desperately ill with typhus and malnutrition from the effects of surviving Auschwitz and Belson.

I had a week only before my unit moved on into the heart of Germany to eradicate completely this malicious virus from humanity. The doctor gave her just a small chance of survival, but promised they would try to keep me informed of any changes in her condition.

On the second of June 1945, I received a message from the doctor in the camp. I opened it slowly, fearing the worst, and read it to myself. "Rose sends her love and is in a hospital in Paris recovering." No words could adequately describe my feelings; it was as if I had awoken from a nightmare.

On the second of September 1945, the war ended and I returned to Paris. Rose and I were the only survivors of both our families.

Bev was in tears, and I was trying to control my emotions. We took Serge out to the reception. "Let me introduce you to Rose, my wife of sixty-two years!" I shook her hand and saw the numbers indelibly burnt onto her left arm. I kissed her on the cheek and said, "It's an honour to meet you. I feel as though I have known you for a long time." Serge smiled at me then with tears in his eyes hugged me and Bev.

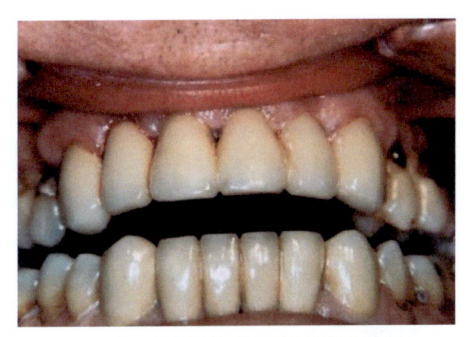

THE NEW LOOK SERGE

THE LONG SLEEP

My name is Colin. Manchester City had just won the premiership, I was happy. It was the most beautiful summer's day, June 2012. The road was clear and I had just reached the top of a long, steep hill that was lined with statuesque trees in their greenest finery. I changed gears on my bicycle anticipating an easy freewheeling ride down. The air was fresh and warm, life was good and I was filled with an almost ecstatic feeling of wellbeing.

I heard the motorbike behind me. Then it was as if I had been hit by a train. I heard a distant voice, "The motorcyclist is dead," and then the whirl of a helicopter and blackness.

More than a dream but less than reality, there I was in a room filled with unrecognisable faces, who almost in unison chanted, *"We are the committee."* I didn't feel dead but thought maybe I was in-between states of existence. *"You are in the blue area, and we have an important mission for you. You must take this letter down to the red area, and under no circumstances must you open it."*

Now at this time I had no memory of life and so assumed that this was a normal request from, well, wherever I was. "How do I get to the red area?" was my obvious request.

"You will soon see, but it will be two weeks before you can go." Then there I was in a sleek soft warm and safe place; some kind of opening and I felt myself being pushed out.

Strange, I thought. Two weeks passed as if time didn't exist. Even stranger was that I had a surreal feeling that I was born two weeks late.

"Ah, you are going to the red zone," uttered the voice. Now I was alone on a bus being driven by a baby that smiled at me, talked and said, "Do you remember what we did with that dirty nappy, and how it landed in the cornflakes? What about all those nights screaming because, well because we could! How about the teddy bear in the toilet?" Did these things happen? I do not know. Then the committee appeared and after discussion, replied in unison, *"Not guilty, he was just a baby."*

All time merged into an instant. The bus drove on but now driven by a child about seven-years-old, looking the image of myself. *"We had a fun childhood in the main,"* the driver declared and continued, *"Mum bathing us every Sunday, then suddenly screaming for our dad. Mum in a state of shock as it seemed we must have had our first erection, maybe she felt we were a little advanced sexually."*

I was spurred into remembering scraps of memory from that age, Mum in hospital whilst Dad did his best to make us breakfast, but the Weetabix was unfortunately disposed of down the toilet. Bonfires kept going for days. I was a bit of a pyrotechnic, and on one occasion used a match to light up the dark area under the couch. Whoosh! It burst into flames, only for my brother to throw water over it. Ruined I had to admit my actions. *"Not guilty again, he was just acting like a mischievous child,"* the committee chorused.

The bus stopped, and on came all my family; cousins, two brothers and friends from school. The driver who was now about thirteen, seemed delighted, obviously because I was also. It was Christmas, the snow was thick and we found ourselves outside in a field. What fun we were having. Then there was Bernadette, my first girlfriend who introduced me to my first lustful experience, which didn't last long! It was a truly happy memory. In this semi-reality I could almost feel the cold snow and the warmth of her body, only disturbed by disapproving looks from all present. A young girl appeared and I just knew that this was my sister who had died at an early age. I hardly knew Maureen, but to see her face now was the most spiritual experience, but then she was gone and the mists of time obscured her memory from me once again.

Suddenly, everyone left the bus and the driver continued the journey. I was now a full-blown teenager, puberty in full bloom, hormones in charge. I felt the hard belt on my backside, six of the best, as the headmaster of my local grammar school decided that my hair was too long and my shoes dirty. *"You will achieve nothing in this world without tidiness and discipline."* His words stayed with me. As I sat on the bus, I found myself smoking, I'm not sure what, and with a bottle in my other hand. This is fun, I thought!

Some discussion by the committee this time before a verdict of *"Not guilty but on probation"* was read out.

Wow, who is this beauty that just boarded the bus? It was Sarah, my fiancée when I was at medical school. I loved this girl and perhaps would have married her if it wasn't for the affair I had with her mother, Maria, who suddenly appeared late on the bus. An apology was just about to be forthcoming but I was interrupted by Maria introducing me to her grandson who was hiding behind her. Sarah smiled. *"Say hello to your son Colin junior!"* I moved over to them but like shadows they disappeared into the ether. I was sure I could hear mumblings from the committee!

It was as if a troubling cloud enveloped me at this stage and I could see people in white coats. I could not think, I could not speak or move, and I could only cry. This was my nervous breakdown. My depressive state included insomnia, loss of hope, anxiety. It was at this stage that I could see nothing in front of me and considered suicide. I lost all my friends and alienated my family. The only people I spoke to were hallucinations, and they couldn't be bothered answering me. The cause? Stress, relationships or possibly lack of advice? No! Stupidity on my part. I was responsible and irresponsible, no discipline and lack of self-esteem. In hospital, there was Helen, my guardian angel who nursed me back to health. I went back to medical school, started to ride my bike everywhere as a cathartic experience. I finished the course and qualified as a doctor, then immediately went to see Helen; I got down on one knee and proposed. She accepted with no hesitation.

"Oh, what a happy ending," said the committee. *"But no, we are not fooled. Guilty on several counts!"*

Then I was on the bus again, and my eight-year-old son Johnny was there in front of me. *"Can I come riding on my bike with you, Dad?"* I was about to agree, but something prevented me. I explained that I was going to try to ride up a very steep hill and it would be too much for him.

The bus stopped! The driver and I were now in our thirties and as I looked at him it was as if I was looking into a mirror. *"You can get off now, we are in the red Zone,"* he signalled to me. Then the bus had gone. I felt cold now for the first time, and there were distant intangible voices and shadows.

"Do you have a letter for me?" a voice demanded. And there was a man, dressed all in red, but with devilish eyes, almost like a football referee from the future. He took the letter. *"Damnation!"* he blurted out.

"*Aguero scores the winner!*" I suddenly felt euphoric and thought I was cheering, I felt alive?

The committee appeared. "*Well, what's the verdict? He delivered the message and has a good heart. He's made a contribution to people's lives, and deserves a chance. NOT GUILTY!*"

As I came round, I felt cold and my skin prickled but I was smiling. "How long have I been in hospital?"

"You've been in a coma for three weeks!" Helen explained. "You've been in and out of consciousness for the last few days. The doctors said you kept muttering something about Sergio!"

I had a fractured neck vertebra as well as serious back damage, broken ribs and my teeth, well let's leave that for now. After recovery I documented all the memories from my three comatose weeks, but I now suffered depression and was not fit enough to return to work.

As soon as I was able, I went to see my dentist, Bernard. To say he was shocked with my appearance was a real understatement. "Colin you've done a lot of damage, but that's why you're here and we will do our best to put you back together."

He had lost many of his front teeth and some on the right-hand side posteriors. In a case like this there could be several options — a removable denture, implants to restore the missing teeth, a fixed bridge which would involve crowning the existing teeth, already restored or damaged. One could even do nothing as an option. We took impressions and my technical support mounted them on an articulator which showed the position of the upper and lower teeth. In this way we were able to assess the best option for him.

After explaining all the various advantages and disadvantages, Colin decided on a fixed bridge. This was completed over three visits of preparation, try-in and then final cementation. After all the checks, we revealed the final result. He was in tears exclaiming how he now felt able to face the world, and his patients again. He was so excited that he was about to leave the surgery when I reminded him that we had not yet cemented the bridge permanently into position. We all laughed. That could had been interesting!

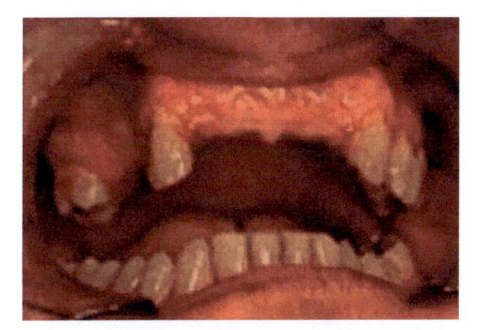

THE OLD COLIN

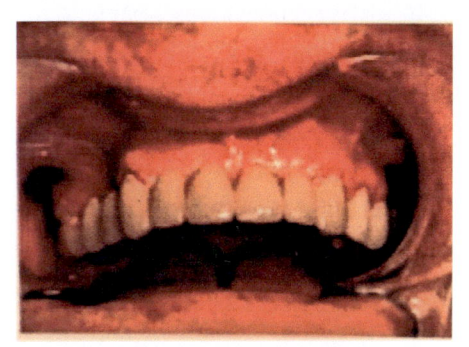

THE NEW COLIN

A LITTLE BOY'S TALE

Children can sometimes be an absolute pleasure to treat, or they can be so frightened by past experiences that any treatment can become almost impossible. We can have television in the surgery, videos and radio distractions and these are really good for creating a relaxing atmosphere, but a nervous child, possibly made to feel worse by stories and anecdotes from other children, and their parents, may not respond to any of these distractions. Our best results came from endeavouring to tell stories to the children which stimulated their imagination, and if they needed several appointments they would often look forward in anticipation to the continuing tale, as we carried on with treatment.

Jimmy was seven-years-old, from a fractured family. His father had left when he was very young and his mother had various medical issues which prevented her from being able to look after him. His grandparents, Carole and Kenneth were caring for him. When we first saw him, we were disturbed by the degree of decay and general neglect in his mouth. A child at this age would have a mixed dentition of first and second teeth, depending on eruption times. Jimmy had four back first permanent molars present which erupt behind the last first (milk) teeth. He also had four lower permanent incisors, and two on the top jaw. All of these permanent teeth were decayed and the remaining first teeth were in a worse condition. Where to begin?

He came into the surgery clutching a small dishevelled teddy bear that had seen better days. Carole, his grandmother, explained that he would take the teddy everywhere with him and it seemed to give him an element of security. He was frightened, shivering, and looked as though he was ready to just run out at the first opportunity. I showed him the examination mirror and demonstrated how we would use it on his teddy bear to count teeth. "What's his name?" I asked. No reply.

We spent twenty minutes showing him how to clean his teddy's teeth, and then with a little persuasion demonstrated on his teeth. He was given a new toothbrush and some special fluoride paste to use, which hopefully would arrest any further decay. "Can you ask your granny to write down what you and teddy eat between now and your next appointment?" Granny nodded in agreement. "Next time I will tell you a story about a little boy your age and his blanket." Jimmy and his granny left the surgery, but on his way out he turned saying, "I call him Ted." A beginning, I thought.

They returned a week later and as I looked at the diet sheet, I could see why his teeth were in such poor condition. A high sugar diet yes, but it was not just the quantity, but the number of times during the day that he had sugary drinks. Here was the cause. Jimmy looked up at me with a pathetic but less frightened face, as if awaiting his fate.

"Jimmy, today I would like to paint some special paste on your teeth and it has a very nice taste to it. Whilst I'm doing this I will tell you about Ben a boy of about your age who had a blanket which kept him safe and secure. He went to sleep with it and took it everywhere with him." Jimmy clutched his teddy closer to his face.

One day Ben was out walking with his granny and granddad and of course the pet dog, Pinky. They had a lovely stroll in the park and Ben played with Pinky having great fun throwing sticks for her to collect.

At this point I started to clean his teeth with a small brush and paint them with the fluoride varnish. The idea being that this can help to harden the enamel.

When Ben returned to his grandparents' house, he suddenly started to cry. "I've lost my blanket". He was very upset, so they all went off to try and find it. It was no use and even Pinky, a very special dog, couldn't find it. Ben wouldn't eat his tea and that night he was heard crying in bed. All he kept repeating was, 'I want my little blanket back.'

Now Pinky, as I said before, was a very special dog. Early in the morning she quietly crept out through the back door and met all the other dogs in the area that were his friends. "Look, I've got a problem," barked

Pinky. "Ben's lost his blanket and if we don't find it I am very worried what may happen to him".

"Hmm," growled Albert the Alsatian. "Leave it to me and I will organise a search party." This he did, and all the dogs went off, sniffing and poking their noses here, there and everywhere. But no, they could not find it."

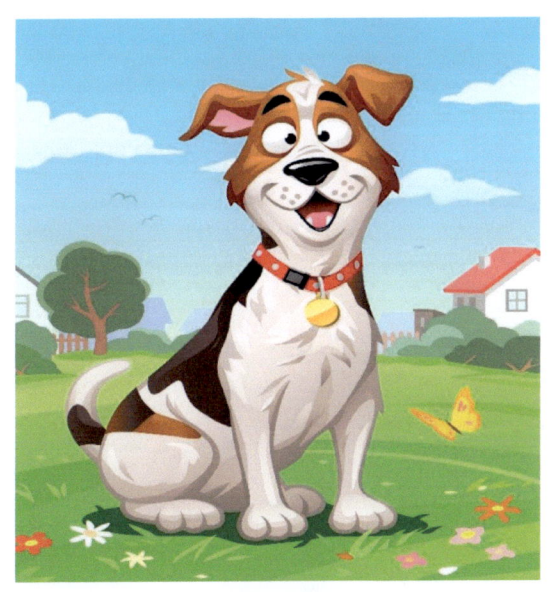

PINKY

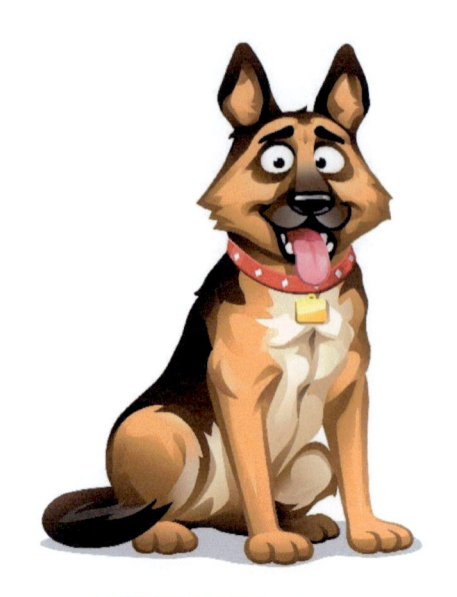

ALBERT THE ALSATIAN

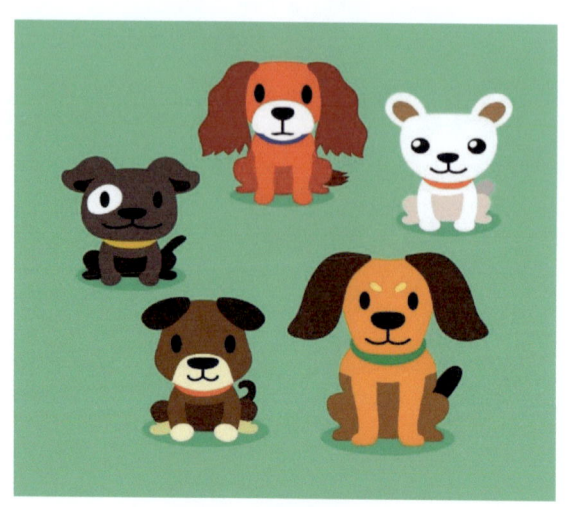

PINKY'S FRIENDS

"Now Jimmy, I'm just going to put some special cement in some of your teeth to try to stop them from hurting in the future." This was a temporary measure but could stop the decay and act as an early filling. Very carefully and without any injections, I gently removed some decay from as many teeth as I could, then put in a little filling material. To my surprise, Jimmy suddenly turned around to me and asked, "Did he find his blanket?" I explained that I would continue the story at the next appointment, but that he must reduce his sugary food intake. Although not animated in his conversation, I thought that Jimmy was perhaps coming out of his shell. I explained to Granny that diet was the key here to avoid extractions, which would be traumatic for him.

"Well Jimmy, how have you been? Have you been taking more care of your teeth?" I enquired, on his next visit to see me. He was a little sheepish but said he had tried and that Ted had helped him. There had been some improvement and so I decided to continue with the oral hygiene instructions, with a little help from my hygienist. Whilst she continued with the treatment, the story unfolded!

Pinky had to think about what to do to find the blanket. Ben was upset, withdrawn and would not play with her. She decided that she needed more help and went outside to find Robbie the Rabbit and his family. "Robbie, I need your help," she pleaded and explained what had happened. The rabbit family was very understanding and decided that they would look in all the holes and burrows in the area to try to find the blanket.

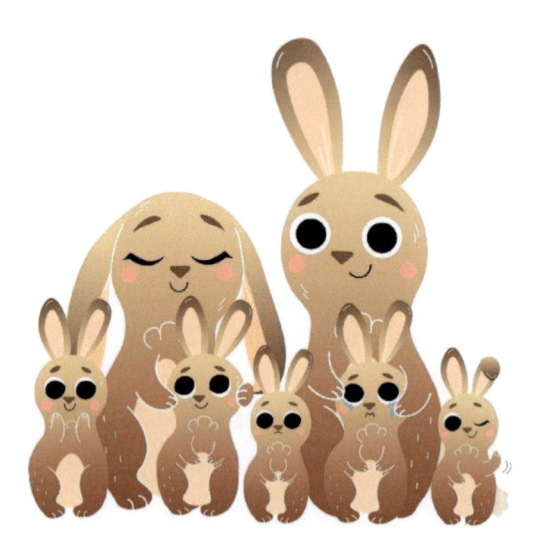

ROBBIE AND FAMILY

They searched all day and into the evening. They found two odd shoes, a hat, an old sandwich but nothing else. Pinky was very upset. "We need some flying help." The rabbits agreed, and went off to find Meggie Magpie and her family. They shouted up to her nest until they flew down to see the rabbits, who explained the problem.

"Right, at first light our squadron will be out in the sky on the lookout for the blanket," Meggie decided.

MEGGIE

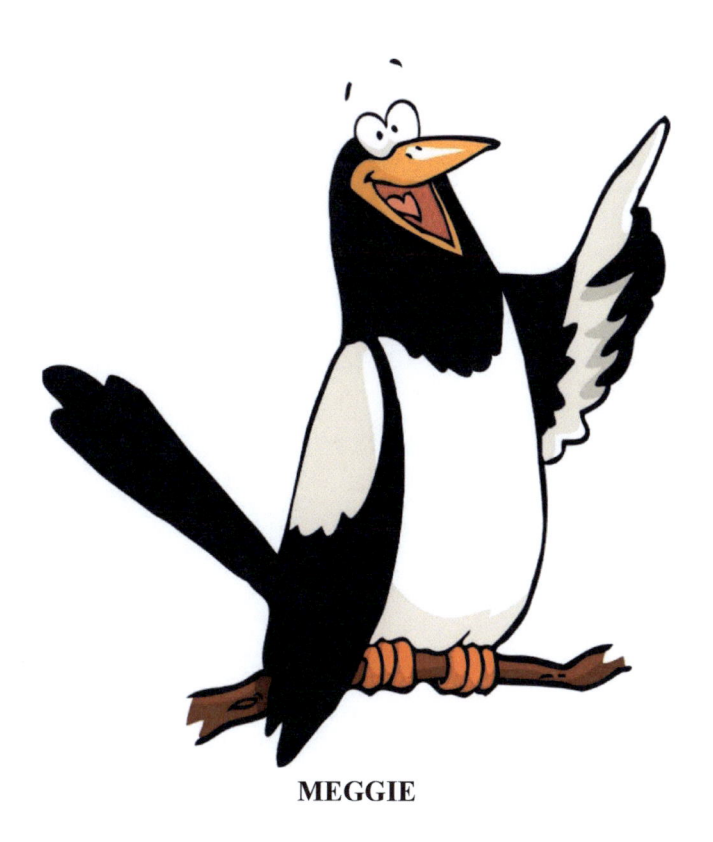

So off they went to search the park from the sky. Well, they found some nice juicy worms for breakfast, some yummy lettuce in a garden for a midmorning snack and some scones on a table they thought were not wanted! But no blanket. Pinky was not going to give up, and wanted to continue the search overnight, but who could see in the dark? "Ollie owl" she excitedly exclaimed and went to find him just before he woke up.

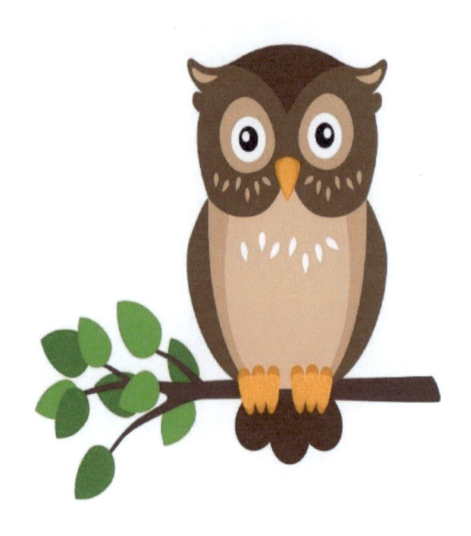

OLLIE OWL

"Ollie, I need your help!" Pinky explained. Ollie said that he twoooooould try to find it for them and promised to search all night.

We had finished treatment for the day and Jimmy had listened attentively. Not only that, he had not been concerned about the procedure. "Next week I am going to put some more fillings in and then we can give you a break for three months."

He jumped off the chair, still clutching Ted and smiled. "Will you be here to finish the story?"

"Of course, I will," and felt a lump in my throat.

On his final appointment I explained that I was going to use some local anaesthetic so it would not hurt at all. He was obviously apprehensive but I first applied a special cream which smelled of bubble gum. "That's nice," he smiled. Because of the surface anaesthetic, I was able to inject a little articaine, to numb up one tooth which had more decay. I very gently cleaned out the cavity with a slow drill, virtually noiseless but with a little vibration. Jimmy was fine and so before I completed the filling, I continued the story.

"Ollie flew all night scanning the ground. He found treats for breakfast, lunch and supper. Then just as it was getting light, he caught sight of something hidden at the edge of a field. 'Twoooooould you believe it? I see it, the blanket!' It was just as described, a small white crocheted square with Ben's name on it. He was so excited, but it was getting light and he had to get it to Meggie as soon as possible. Ollie flew to her nest, stopping on the way for a little snack of an old apple. 'Meggie, I've found it!' tweeted Ollie.

Meggie the Magpie was a little tired and hungry, so before flying off to find Robbie Rabbit, she stopped for another nice juicy worm and a big crust of bread. 'That's better,' and then off she went to find the rabbits.

Meggie found Robbie who was busy munching some vegetables he had found in a garden. 'I'll take it straight away to Albert the Alsatian,' so off he hopped. Robbie searched and searched for him, then suddenly he saw him at the gate of his house. 'Albert, I've got the blanket!' the rabbit squealed.

'I sniffed that there may have been progress,' Albert growled and took the blanket from Robbie who looked a little frightened. 'Don't worry, I've not had my breakfast yet but I'll take it straightaway to find Pinky.' Leaping over fences and weaving through gardens, off he went. Then there she was sitting at the front door of Ben's house. She was so excited. The two dogs did a little dance and had a quick nuzzle; they had always been good friends. Pinky was so happy She rushed through the back door and up to Ben's bedroom where he was still asleep. Carefully placing the blanket on the bed she realised it was very dirty. Off she went and woke up granny, whimpered and showed her the blanket. "You are a clever dog, aren't you? But it will need a quick wash." Within half an hour the blanket was washed, dried and put near where Ben could see it.

Pinky waited at the bedside until he woke up. "Oh Pinky, you found my blanket. You are the cleverest dog in the whole world." Ben nuzzled the blanket and was over the moon, so much happier. Pinky wanted to explain that she had had a lot of help, but took the credit for it, sensibly!

I finished the treatment and told Jimmy he would feel a little numb in his mouth for a few hours. He jumped off the chair, and didn't seem concerned. I explained to his grandmother Carole that he had to be very careful with his diet and tooth cleaning. She hugged Jimmy. "He's a different boy now, really looking after his teeth so much more. We have banned the fizzy drinks and reduced the frequency of his sugar intakes," Carole explained.

Then Jimmy who had only shown affection to his teddy suddenly ran over to me and gave me a hug. "Mr Dentist," he said, "will you tell me another story like that when I return?"

I was truly touched and replied, "Of course I will!" I turned to my nurse Bev, no pressure there then!

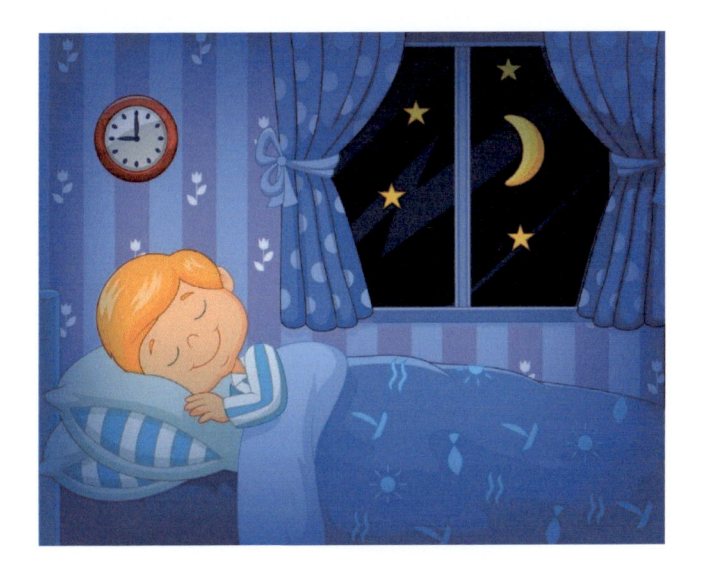

SEXUAL HEALING?

Mike qualified at Dental School with me and we were good friends, sharing good times as well as bad. She was the 'Casanova' of our group, six feet tall, blond hair swept back and with a physique like a body builder. He was immensely popular and exuded confidence and self-esteem. As we progressed through our course, it became apparent that he was having several relationships with nurses, and one member of the staff. No problem there, but I noticed this was having a really bad effect on his mental state, combined with a sudden aggressive attitude towards people who knew him. After we qualified, we kept in touch, I was married and Mike was in and out of relationships, none of which made him happy or even content. Then for ten years we lost contact.

When I saw him again it was as a patient coming to see me for some extensive treatment. He had lost a front tooth and hated the denture he had to wear. He wanted an implant and knew that I had started to provide this treatment. Being unsure where to go he decided it had to be to somebody he knew. Mike had changed. That brash almost over-confidence had gone, and together with lost weight and thinning hair, he was no longer the figure I had admired and remembered.

Implants can be used to replace single or multiple teeth lost, and are completed usually in stages. In Mike's case, from trauma to the mouth, he had lost his upper incisor. Quite how he lost it was an embarrassment to him but he promised to tell me after treatment was complete. After the initial x-rays and a CT scan, which gives a three-dimensional image of the area, I organised my oral surgeon to place the implant in position with a local anaesthetic. After a period of four months, he then opened up the implant so that I was able to complete the restorative stages. This involved impressions and the construction of an abutment screwed into the implant head. On this the crown, made in bonded porcelain to gold, was fitted. The end result was as good as new.

"Now Mike, how did you lose the tooth?" He looked sheepishly at me and we arranged to have dinner and catch up. "I warn you, the story I am going to tell you is frightening and true. My life as you can see has changed and you will understand why," he confided in a very serious voice.

Mike looked at me and I detected a tear in his eye as he began to explain the story of his last ten years.

"When we all qualified as dentists, life seemed easy. Untroubled at first until reality hit. It was the pressure of running my own surgery, acquired after I had been invited to take over from a colleague who had died suddenly.

A large Scotch at night helped, then a nip at lunchtime, and before I knew it, I was drinking before surgery. I thought I could control it, which I did at first, but I soon realised that I was in trouble. My personal life was no better; I had relationships that were meaningless, that gave me no lasting pleasure. Sex became a drug as I struggled with my addiction, and I used women as receptacles for my own amusement. My life seemed to have no direction or aim. On a rare visit to see my ageing parents, suggestions were made to me to seek medical advice or I would risk losing everything. It's hard to explain but addiction is not just a habit, it's a need in order to function. I realised it was time to make an effort to change direction in my life, or give up completely, a frightening thought that instilled an overwhelming feeling of panic in me. But not now, maybe some other time. My current girlfriend, Christine, had everything. She was clever, mischievous, kind and sensual, but I had treated her badly. She had talked about cementing our relationship, but I said I had not yet met a woman I could live with. This I could see was like a dagger to her heart. I felt nothing. Plenty more available women.

"I was in the waiting room of the psychologist and sex therapist recommended by my GP. It was a soothing room, furnished minimally but warm with a scattering of books and magazines aimed at distracting clients.

One book caught my eye, *A Christmas Carol* by Charles Dickens. This was my favourite book as a child and it conjured up images that I can still recall of snowy Christmases at home with my family, a sumptuous turkey dinner and presents."

"Please come in Michael," invited a statuesque woman who guided me into her consulting room. She introduced herself as Julia Morley, but it was her eyes that transfixed me. It was as if her gaze had pinned me to my chair, I could not move. She had an almost surreal appearance, beautiful and hypnotic, and her words barely registered with me. I found myself blurting out my troubles, all my disasters, the innumerable women that I had used and discarded.

Then the consultation ended. "I will see you again, soon," Julia explained. "After I have given some thought to your case."

I left feeling strange, nervous and in awe of that ethereal experience, but after a few glasses of my favourite Scotch at home, I put the disturbing events behind me. I was convinced that I was capable of running my own life without outside help or interference. "Humbug!" I laughed uncontrollably. Damn it, I can sort this out myself. Brave words which were my undoing, because ultimately I could not.

I was having a disturbed night trying to sleep, often the case after improving the economy of Scotland. It must have been the early hours, I wasn't sure, when I heard footsteps on the stairs leading to my room. I was terrified. I listened hardly daring to breathe. Nothing, a dream and I lay back on the pillow. "Hello Michael, remember me?"

My eyes tried to close but could not. I wanted to breathe but struggled and I wanted to wake up but couldn't. There in front of me was Julia Morley. No this could not be. "How did you get in? You aren't real". Then a hand touched my arm and gently grasped hold. "Michael, let us look at some of the girls and women you have known in the past, then tell me your thoughts." "Not a bloody chance," I heard myself scream. But to no avail.

Then there I was, looking at pornography in school, my friends avidly taking in the exotic images. The scene changed to my classroom. "What happens next when you take a bite of apple?" our biology teacher asked.

In confident mood I answered, "You masturbate it, sir." Complete silence! "I think you mean masticate, don't you?" The class collapsed in laughter; my embarrassment was complete.

Suddenly I was with my first girlfriend, fumbling, trying to put on a condom. She looked down and burst into laughter. "It looks like a frozen sausage." My confidence dissipated, much like the erection.

Julia led me further; there I was in the back seat of my father's car, satisfying my testosterone-fuelled urges with sixteen-year-old Jennifer. No contraception, I'll take a chance. "Remember her, Michael? You never saw Jennifer again, despite many calls from her explaining her situation. She had a termination but she never fully recovered from that trauma. But what did you care?" Plenty more available women.

Suddenly I was back in Dental School. "The nurses adored you Michael. They helped you in your work and you conjured up ways to repay them with a complete lack of respect, affection and loyalty." There was Jean in front of me, large as life. I told her I loved her and was invited to meet her parents. A wonderful warm home, a sister, brother and adoring parents. "Yes Michael, this could have been perfect, had it not been for you having an affair with her mother, being found out, causing mayhem, havoc and divorce." Destruction complete.

"Just receptacles for your own amusement." Julia stared at me with cold eyes and pointed a finger at me. "By now you had what you'd always wanted, your own surgery. But did you care about your predecessor, his ideas, the patients he cared for? No, you arrogantly carried on in a cesspool of selfishness, of your own making.

"Can you develop these x-rays?" I heard myself saying to my manageress, Maria. Then I was stroking her thighs and breasts. "Let's make love before we start work?"

She pushed me away. "Make love? You don't know the meaning of the word. Having sex is all you understand, no feeling, no emotion. That's not enough for me. I will be leaving at the end of the week." No loss

I thought. She was barely adequate in and out of the bedroom.

"And so, Michael, another person who cared for you but did you care for her? Did you show any concern or affection? No, plenty more available women. Did you know she was pregnant with your child?"

"What!" I heard myself exclaim in horror.

"Yet you always found solace with escorts. Did you feel the highs and lows of an orgasm helped you? Did you feel that if you paid for a sexual relationship, it meant you had to give even less back? Was it this 'pay as you go' that appealed? They didn't ask for any emotional attachment. Did it ever occur to you that they were using you as nothing more than a source of income, and laughing at you?" Those words hurt me and hit home, and I recall that after I'd been particularly abusive to one woman, it was her right hook that caused me to lose the front tooth. A tooth for a tooth, *c'est la vie*.

Then I was sitting in my office before surgery, taking my usual Valium tablet washed down with a whisky. I was near the bottom I could tell. Last patient of the day, a lovely woman who made it obvious I could see more of her if I wanted. I couldn't refuse. Helen would come back to the surgery late after everybody had left. At first there was an intense excitement that I once thought might develop into a more substantial liaison, but no, the alcohol and sedatives were having a bad effect. My libido had gone and I became abusive towards her on her last visit, telling her I didn't want to see her again.

Christine appeared and I felt a sudden burst of relief, a face I knew and trusted, a face that I had neglected and a soul that I had trodden underfoot. All she wanted was to show her love and concern for me. I could see the genuine feeling in her eyes, turning to pity. What had I thrown away? I was on the edge, between what I knew to be good and wholesome and what I had become.

Julia approached me again. "You have managed to destroy every relationship offered to you, ruined lives and families with your inability to control your actions. Was it because of all those times people laughed at you when you were a boy growing up and coming to terms with your sexuality? Well, you are a man now, but let's look at what effect these actions could have on your future."

My parents were there in front of me, not smiling but with stern looks. "Just look at yourself in the mirror. You've lost your friends, said goodbye to Christine who loved you dearly. You reek of alcohol and cigarettes, look used and burnt out." My mother never minced her words.

"You need to trace your sexual partners over the past four weeks," said the doctor. Oh no! Was I really in the Venereal Disease clinic? "You have a purulent penile discharge, probably caused by gonorrhoea. I will give you an antibiotic injection and you must return in two weeks for further tests. I think we can discount syphilis but I want to be sure." The sample tube inserted into my penis was beyond painful, more like a hot needle being pushed in. Was this my punishment, my just desserts? Was it too late to change?

"Your fitness to practise has been questioned and an accusation has been made by a patient that on several occasions you had sexual relations with her in your surgery. This is a most serious complaint, unfortunately confirmed by a member of your staff. If upheld I have to tell you that YOUR NAME WILL BE REMOVED FROM THE DENTAL REGISTER". A lightning bolt hit me. My face burned and my heart thudded in my chest. I could not speak. I knew I was guilty and had to take the consequences. This was the General Dental Council and I was confronted by a group of my peers, ghostly leering figures who were rightly ready to deprive me of my livelihood, and worse, a possible criminal conviction. No way out. My apology would fall on deaf ears, the group would be unmoved. Take my punishment.

Julia was there again. "Is this really my future, could it be changed?" Then a funeral, my family gathered around. Christine, Maria with a small child, staff members and you Bernard, you were there saying a few words over the coffin. Blackness.

Was this heaven or hell?

I'm back in the surgery lying flat on the dental chair, nobody there, but I can't move, my hands and feet bound tight to the unit. I struggled but couldn't move, fear and panic gripped me like a thick fog. Then a voice, Maria, then many faces, Jean, Helen, with those familiar girls and women I had known whose names I had long forgotten. So, this was it, my ultimate demise, surrounded by all the people I had used, all the relationships I had ruined, all the chances missed. Accept my fate. But what are they waiting for?

Julia appeared with something in her hand, a scalpel, scissors? I couldn't tell, but fear gripped me again as eager hands pulled at my trousers until all was laid bare. So, this was what awaited me. I closed my eyes and waited for the inevitable cut, my screams, blood and laughter.

Julia carefully flashed the scalpel blade in front of my eyes, my reflection in the blade showed a face beyond fear. Salty tears poured out. Visions of my childhood drifted in front of me, I felt emotions exude from primeval depths. She took the blade and cut the straps holding me. A euphoria filled me with a happiness that I had never felt, and I leaned forward to embrace her. "I can change," I spluttered in a frenzy of relief and expectation.

Julia smiled. "I know you can, but if you don't I can see you again." With a flash of the blade and a smile she was gone.

In bed, a dream? No, something in-between imagination and reality? There next to the bed was the answer, a scalpel.

Dressed and ready for the day I had planned. Straight to see Christine, I'll surprise her. I took my mother's engagement ring, given to me in the vain hope that one day I might find the right person to pass it on to. Christine looked beautiful. It was as if I was seeing her in a new and different light. "Well, you look as though you've had a really rough night and just seen a ghost," she joked, with a twinkle in her eye that disarmed me completely. Even that mysterious comment was not going to stop me. "Marry me!" I pleaded. Before I could get an answer, I pushed the ring onto her finger.

"Wow, what's caused this sudden change of heart?"

I smiled, now relaxed as if within me a new spirit had emerged. I bent down on one knee and explained. "Because for the first time in my life I realise and know that I love you and that I will be a better human being with you by my side. You are the only one for me." With tears in her eyes, she accepted.

I was completely honest with Christine. We talked about the way I had behaved, the way forward, and our wedding plans. No room for error in this relationship. We agreed that I should see Maria, to make my peace with her.

On a bright sunny day, I arrived at her house, and with trepidation I rang the doorbell. There was Maria with a small boy. Stunned to see me, she stared unblinking, turned to the child and spoke gently.

"Andrew, say hello to your father." I see him again whenever possible. I have tried to be a good father to him, although part time, which suited Maria perfectly. Over the next few months, we became, not a family, but good friends.

"Bernard, all the things in the dream were true, except what could happen in the future, I can change them and I will." Mike kindly insisted on paying for the meal, and was assisted by a rather attractive waitress who smiled at him whilst clearing cutlery from our table. Suddenly light caught a knife. He stared at the image in the reflection, visibly paled, turned to me and spoke. "I want you to be my best man."

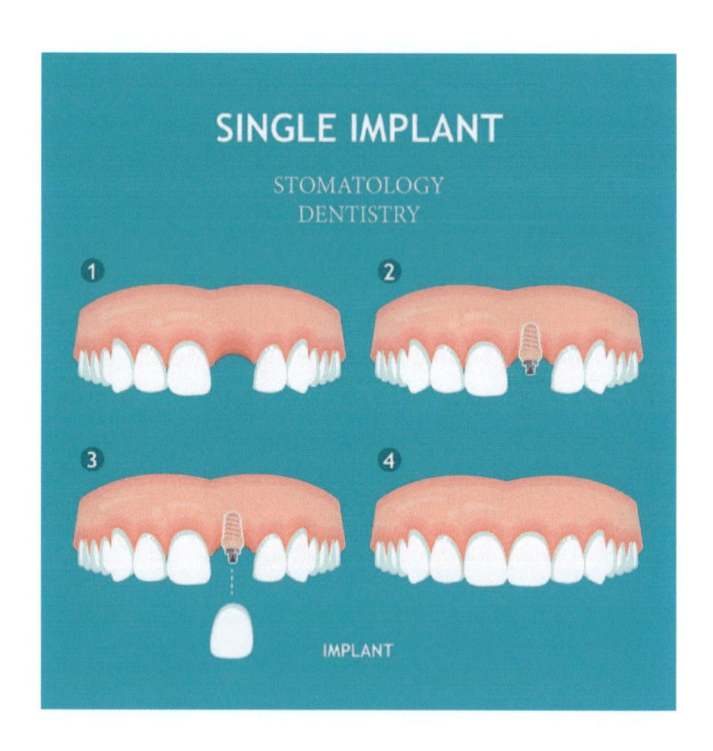

The implant is placed into the bone where the tooth is missing, (1). Once integration around the implant has taken place, (2), an abutment support is made to fit into it, (3), and then the crown is constructed as above, (4).

BOOK 2
THE NURSES' TALES

PIP'S STORY: THE ACCIDENTAL SAMARITANS

Not bleak mid-winter but not far off. A freezing snowy dark December morning, black ice on the roads, cars skidding all over and the path up to the surgery door like a slalom event. I struggled to get through the door and into the waiting room, hoping I could thaw my hands out and prepare for the day. As I entered, the change of climate was almost tropical. The storage heaters had worked — not always the case — the television was on and a full waiting room was glued to the morning news. Better still was the pervading aroma of fresh toast from the kitchen. Hot tea, buttered crumpets and I was ready for the day.

A normal surgery list, patients in pain, a child who had slipped on the ice and damaged his front tooth, a denture to be fitted and sundry crowns on nervous patients. The mood was always sombre when they came in for treatment but on the way out a change, a smile and a thank you. This always perked us up and we thought we had completed a satisfactory morning of sorting the nation's teeth.

As I walked to check the waiting room at the end of the session there was one gentleman still there, asleep in the corner where he would not have been easily noticed. A wizened, thin and dishevelled man, a torn coat with missing buttons and his rough fingers clutching a woollen hat. He suddenly woke up and looked at me. Not wanting to frighten him I enquired if he had an appointment. His reply filled me with sadness and concern.

"I'm sorry," he mumbled. "I was just walking past feeling so cold when I saw the lights on in the surgery. It looked warm and cosy and was the only house that had no frost on the windows, so I walked in and sat down. I felt so comfortable I must have dozed off."

He could barely stand up and was about to leave when I asked him if he would like a hot drink before he left. The smile on his face was like the sun coming out from behind a black cloud. By this time the rest of the staff had come to see our stowaway and determined to help, they prepared a mug of tea and a plate of biscuits for him. His mood changed and he became cheerful and animated. He left the surgery, certainly in a better frame of mind, telling us all his name, Terry.

The following day was even worse weather. The patients poured into the surgery in a constant stream. Terry was among the first, and he became almost at home in the waiting room, telling the strangers snippets of his life story. "I was an orphan," he explained. "My first memory was of a row of children, no parents, nobody to pick you up when you cried, and worst of all no idea of what the future held or who with. One of the boys, about my age had toothache. There was no dentist and so the nurse in charge prised the offending tooth out with a fork."

"Er, Terry, that's not good for business," reacted the receptionist, much to everyone's amusement. "I went from foster home to foster home. Some of the people were lovely, kind and affectionate. Others were the opposite, and it was when I was eleven-years-old that the physical abuse began. Eventually the council put me with a couple in Yorkshire, and it was here that I learnt to become a coal miner, just at the outbreak of war. John and Sheila were perfect, no children of their own, and it seemed that I was unofficially adopted. They looked after me wonderfully. John was in the merchant navy, but sadly died when his ship was torpedoed. That only left Sheila who was in poor health and struggled to keep the house and myself in one piece. Eventually she had to move in with her sister and I was left to fend for myself. As I was too young to be called up, in my teens I continued to work down the mines, doing my share for the war effort."

Terry had become a fixture in the surgery, with some patients missing their turn for treatment because he was at an interesting point in his story. "I married Mary at a small church in the village. We had a small rented house and stayed there for twenty years until my dear wife died. We had no children and I was alone again. Those twenty years were my happiest. Then the mine closed and since then my life has been one of wandering the country, hospital visits for my lungs and work wherever I could."

He used to spend time with our denture technician Bart on the top floor, taking him tea and doing errands for him. On one memorable and snowy occasion, Bart and Terry came downstairs chuckling away, covered in snow and looking like a pair of abominable snowmen. "There's a hole appeared in the roof," Bart exclaimed, right on top of where we were sitting. Terry added, "but the job had to be finished." There was abundant laughter all round, a wonderful moment.

As we were due to close before Christmas, we managed to find Terry some more clothes and put together a basket of food. We said our goodbyes and watched him cross the road and go into the church opposite the surgery. We thought that was strange.

We were back at work after the Christmas break but with no improvement in the weather. Where's Terry? we wondered. No sign of our adopted staff member.

Two weeks later we received a letter from the hospital which is very close to us. There was a covering letter from them saying that a man called Terry Jones of no fixed abode had died after being found in the church opposite the surgery. He had given our address for the letter. There were no next of kin or friends to be contacted.

I opened the letter and sobbed uncontrollably.

Terry's letter:
As my life ends and I review my days,
Some deeds become clear in the gathering haze.
That you took me in when I was stricken,
Will make the angels smile as I go to heaven.
As I pass from this world to the next,
My final memories will be the best.
A heartfelt thanks for all your care,
God bless you, don't change, don't dare.
The world is full of uncaring and blindness,
And needs more of your compassion and kindness.
Thank you, Terry.

SUE'S STORY. THE ACCIDENTAL STABLES:

You know the feeling! You wake up, dress and put on makeup. A beautiful spring day, the sun beaming through the windows, you are not working and have a day to yourself. Euphoria! Then the phone rings. It's the surgery. Two staff off with illness, could I come in and help out? Depression! "Get a taxi," the boss says. "There are no buses because of the strike. We need you as soon as possible."

Not the best day to order a taxi, a two-hour wait at least. They cannot cope with the extra demand. Next time I have a day off and I wake up feeling on top of the world, I will wait for the phone to ring before I make any plans for the day. What can I do? I can't walk to work, it's too far. Time to think.

Coffee in my hand, staring out at the field opposite my house. There's the love of my life! My horse Merry, happily munching on the grass. At least he will get a day off, I thought. Or will he?

They do say necessity is the mother of invention. I wonder! I gaze across at him. To this day I am sure he nodded his head from side to side as if to say, "No way!"

It was the only form of transport I had. No buses, no taxis and nobody nearby to help me out with a car. I was not on any train route so this was it. I took a bag with my surgery gear, a saddle and everything else I needed for my horse, then walked over to the field. Merry who had seen me, trotted off in the opposite direction. My secret weapon, two apples shown to him prompted him to turn back towards me.

Fully saddled up, helmet on, off I went. The safest way I thought whilst in heavy traffic, was to stay as close to the pavement as I was able. Merry had been out on the road many times and took no prisoners from irate drivers. Still, I was making good progress, weaving my way through the cars, occasionally nudging a wing mirror, much to the annoyance of one driver. "Hey!" he yelled through his now open window. "What's it like to drive a one horse power vehicle?" The joker and his passengers seemed to be enjoying the spectacle, until Merry deposited the abundant remnants of yesterday's grass over the nearside wing of his car. With a sideways glance towards the now furious driver, we trotted away leaving him trying to remove the steaming manure with his handkerchief.

After forty minutes we arrived at the surgery. Now, I thought, where to park my transport?

Fortunately, we have a side gate at the surgery that leads to a sizable back garden with a substantial grassy area. Ideal, I thought.

Merry settled into his temporary residence readily, munching at the overgrown lawn. Well, I thought, this may save a visit from the gardener. I scuttled in unnoticed, with a cursory thanks for coming in from the boss saying that he would pay for the taxi. Ha! That might cost him more than he imagines.

After getting changed I put on my most professional face and started working with Bernard in the surgery that was adjacent to our "stable." A smile to myself. If Merry stays quiet I may get away with this and no mishaps, although I was sure I could see slight movement through the frosted glass that overlooked our garden.

Our last patient before lunch was a lovely slightly deaf gentleman called Ronald, in his eighties, having his new full dentures fitted. Bernard carefully unwrapped them from the laboratory box and placed them in position in Ronald's mouth. "Well, how do they feel?" asked Bernard with a knowing smile that said they were a very good fit. No reply from our patient. Suddenly Ronald took out an apple from his pocket and started to try out his new teeth, this being the ultimate test of security. Oh no! I thought. But before I could stop him, he munched into the apple. My heart began to pound and I could feel myself perspiring in anticipation. I looked out towards the garden. Too late. There loomed the shadow of Merry tapping on the slightly open window. Then with one push my transport for the day pushed his head and neck into the surgery in an attempt to seize the apple.

Ronald never heard a thing! Then he shouted, "The teeth work perfectly," at the same time thrusting his hand holding the apple in the air in triumph. With a deft swipe Merry took the much-travelled fruit that seemed to be offered freely, romping away to the back of the garden before any action to stop him.

Bernard: What the…?

Ronald: Where's my bloody apple gone?

Me: Erm… I'll just go and get lunch ready!

BEV'S STORY: THE ACCIDENTAL DELIVERY?

Domiciliary visits are never easy. We have to pack a bag with everything we will need, often to take impressions or do examinations. We were due to go to an extremely good residential home in Sale, in Greater Manchester. I had packed the bag and we were ready to go, but there was a problem. Being seven months pregnant and finding it a little difficult to drive over longer distances, it was decided that Bernard would do the driving in my car, a Ford Escort. This was to be my last week in work before maternity leave.

The route took us onto the M602 then over the notorious Barton Bridge on what is now the M60 which spans the Manchester Ship Canal, both great engineering feats. I was determined to complete this last domiciliary visit before leave, and we had three sets of impressions to take.

It was one of those special spring mornings in 1996, when nature was at its best, when we were all feeling refreshed after a long hard winter, and I was looking forward to the birth and a few weeks' respite. Remember though, I loved my job, the independence it brought me and the complete trust that was put in me to run the private surgery. The traffic was as ever heavy and slow, but we had plenty of time so no need to concern ourselves. We were on the M602 and just joining what is now the M60 at the bottom of Barton Bridge. All seemed normal as we moved onto the motorway and stayed on the inside lane.

If you have ever been in an accident, you will know that things sometimes seem blurry and surreal, with images that seem to be outside normal reality. I will describe what happened with no exaggeration or embellishment, because if it had not been for a modicum of luck and some good driving, the outcome could have been so, so different.

There was a bang, and we felt as though a giant hand had pushed us up Barton Bridge. Bernard controlled the car as best he could and kept it on the carriageway. I remember looking over the edge of the bridge into the Ship Canal and thinking we going to end up there.

Suddenly we were free! But then again, another huge crashing sound as this time we were spun around facing the oncoming three lanes of traffic. This was our worst nightmare. We could see what had hit us — a twenty-two-ton milk lorry that could not stop. We were spun round again and at one point faced the Ship Canal. This is it, I thought, over the barrier and try to escape from the water. Fear. No, terror would be closer. I had everything going for me in life, married with a lovely house, career, family and friends. A wonderful job, all to be lost. In those few seconds my life seemed to be put on hold as time stood still. We seemed to move inexorably towards the edge.

Then Bernard regained control while the lorry continued down the hill on the other side of the bridge where it eventually came to a halt. We ended up facing three lanes of stationary traffic and stopped. Relief, no — much, much more. We looked at each other and knew how close we had come to disaster; how sudden unexpected occurrences can change lives. Bernard was horrified and was only concerned about me and my baby.

Then the police arrived. The tow truck turned us round and to my amazement we were able to drive the car to the next exit, with police escort. We spoke to the driver of the milk lorry who claimed that another car had forced him into hitting us. He then admitted that he could not stop due to defective brakes.

We started to laugh, I think just with relief, then the pains started. Not labour pains, it seemed to be more sinister. The police called an ambulance, I needed to be checked over. Was this going to be a premature baby? Had the accident caused more serious problems? I could not bear those thoughts and tried to put them out of my mind. I was whisked to the hospital and examined. Normal heart beat from the baby, not for me though. I felt like my palpitations would be the end of me. Soon though, it settled. No bruises, no marks. Bernard and I were just so pleased to be in one piece.

The car, when we looked at it again was frightening. Every side had been dented and squashed, as if some giant press had just pushed it out of shape.

We were back in the surgery the next day, but for the first hour we just went over and over the accident, thinking was there any way we could have avoided it. What did we do wrong? Nothing. We were just in the wrong place when a fully loaded milk lorry went out of control.

The driver was fined and found guilty of dangerous driving. My car was a complete write-off. Strangely, about three months later we had a call from a person in Ireland who was planning to purchase the car, which he said looked in good condition! He wanted to know if the mileage was genuine. After I explained to him that the car had been severely damaged, he thanked us and said he would not now consider it.

To this day, some twenty-five years later, I have a quiet moment and think what could have happened, but thankfully did not. Whenever I go over the bridge I recall vividly those events, and I'm always relieved when I'm down on the other side.

JEAN'S STORY: THE FLYING FIFTY PENCE (told by the dentist!)

It was one of those nights. I just could not get to sleep, so at three a.m. I started to read my dental journals until I must have nodded off finally.

It still felt like the middle of the night when I was woken by my alarm, on a frosty cold dark morning. You will know exactly what I mean when I say you go to work in the dark and come home, also in the dark. We all seem to be affected by the Seasonally Affected Syndrome (SAD) at this time of year. I cleared the frost off the car then noticed the rather flat tyre. Just what I needed, a perfect start to the day. I managed to drive the car into a position where the tyre could be changed, then decided to go back to bed. But no, my professional conscience took over and I ordered a taxi.

I arrived in the surgery to find the staff struggling to get the heating on which was supposed to start automatically at a certain time of day. Eventually someone decided it would work if the power was switched on!

An auspicious start to the day. But coffee was served, we were getting warmer and the patients seemed to be in jolly moods, possibly because of Christmas looming.

Jean, my nurse is a lovely lady, of Greek Cypriot origin. What this means is that she was one of the best nurses that I'd been blessed to work with. With that dark straight hair and Mediterranean vivacious looks, she was very popular with the patients, well half of them anyway! Jean was always ready to help out in an emergency, and was, because of the way she had been raised, respectful of her position, and those around her. She was however, extremely volatile on occasions, usually when something was troubling her.

Unusually, when she arrived she went straight to the smoking area outside (amazing but we had a dedicated place at that time). Eventually she came into the surgery, said hello and carried on with her duties. No small talk, no how are you today? Just a pervading atmosphere like a volcano getting ready to explode.

Now I wasn't in the best frame of mind and would have appreciated a chat to clear the air and find out what was wrong, but no, I decided it was best to keep the volcano only simmering.

We had seen three patients, but I knew we had a full waiting room, often the case with the NHS. I buzzed through to the receptionist and asked her to send Jean in with next patient. I waited, and waited, eventually ringing through again to find out what was going on.

Enough I thought, I'm tired and feeing very irritable. I never want to keep the patients waiting. Into reception I stormed to find Jean on the phone having what seemed to be a quite animated and friendly conversation. Bluntly and out of character, I said quietly, "Please get off the phone right now."

Back in the surgery I waited, and waited again, then got out of my chair ready for a fight. Jean walked into the surgery with a red face and looking like some lovely Amazon who was about to tear me limb from limb! I stepped back, not anticipating this reaction.

She looked straight at me, took out a fifty pence piece from her pocket, and slammed it down on my desk. "Here's fifty pence for the phone call," she yelled at me.

"I don't want the bloody fifty pence, I want my next patient!" I exclaimed. Now here is a lesson in what not to do. Instead of asking what was wrong and was there anything I could do to help, I picked up the said coin and hurled it at maximum velocity towards the door, fortunately just after she had left the room, not that I noticed. The fifty pence piece unbelievably embedded itself in the wood of the door. Now I'm not violent as a rule and was truly shocked. Then the receptionist rang through to say that I had left the speaker line open. Was there anything she could help with as she and the remaining patients in the waiting room had heard the whole drama? This was said with a casual air of schadenfreude.

I sat down, took a deep breath and tried to compose myself. Jean then trounced into the surgery all smiles with the patient. She moved to whisper in my ear what I thought was an apology, looked at the door and quietly said, "If you move that bloody fifty pence from the door you will have worse than a riot on your hands, you will have a mutiny!"

Later in the day she came in to apologise and explained the personal problems she was having. I felt awful. I was in the wrong and I knew it. We had a hug and both decided that squabbles would never happen again.

"Let's forget about it now," as I went to remove the coin.

"Don't you dare touch it; it stays put." The door has been redecorated twice since that incident, and the fifty pence piece has long gone, but if you look carefully there is a small circle, unpainted in the door as a constant reminder. This has remained to this day and all efforts to erase it have been stopped, proving that 'hell hath no fury like a woman scorned. '

A VIEW FROM BOTH SIDES OF THE PROBE

THE PATIENT

Do you know fear? Well, I will tell you what it feels like. My name is Fiona Peters. I'm twenty- seven years old, married to a wonderful man. We have a lovely home, a dog and my pride and joy, an F-type Jaguar. My husband Tom has no interest in cars and is happy to cycle to work. He does however have an above average libido, or so he tells me. Our sex life is, well let's say way beyond average. He says I'm insatiable which I rather like, it gives me a feeling of, well if you are a woman, you will know what I mean.

I love my job as an estate agent, meeting people, the thrill of closing a deal. I'm afraid of nothing, except one thing — The Dentist.

I've got to have a root treatment and I'm petrified. As soon as the appointment is made, I'm off everything, can't eat, can't drink and any intimacy becomes alien to me, which has been noticed. I'm irritable and can't settle. Going to the surgery is the last thing I think about at night and the first thing I think about when I wake up. I have been told what's involved, and googled it, a mistake! Tiny reamers screwed into the root of my tooth, removal of any remaining nerve. As they go deeper into the tooth, will there be a moment of excruciating pain? The apprehension is unbearable. It becomes an intense, unabating fear of putting myself in his hands, not that I would object if he was not doing my teeth! Will the local anaesthetic be enough? Should I ask him to put more in to be safe?

"Just a little prick in the mouth," he will say, I would definitely settle for that! What if the nerve is still alive? Oh no, I've just gone through a red light on the way to work! This is ridiculous as I try to convince myself that this is a routine visit. No, it's not, it's a root treatment, the wrenching out of a nerve from my tooth! I pull over and start my breathing exercises.

Eventually I arrive at the office and go straight to the lady's loo. As I sit there, I realise that my fear is totally illogical; he has never hurt me before, but then I have never had a root treatment before. So, there is always a first time!

The day of my appointment has arrived, and I'm booked in as the last patient. I can't eat and can't get out of the bathroom. My insides are churning and twisting. I feel sick and my heart's pounding. I walk around the house and find a cigarette, although I haven't smoked for years. I leave it unlit between my lips as a comfort.

I'm in the waiting room. The pervading odour of antiseptic adds to my fear. I'm alone. "Hello Fiona, how are you?" The receptionist Patricia has already sensed my nervousness and is doing her best to relax me. Not working.

"I'm good thanks," I mutter, "and you?"

"Don't ask. My boyfriend has just asked me to move in with him, and he says I can bring my dogs with me. Trouble is he lives with his parents and he wants me to stay there. The lack of privacy would not make for a romantic atmosphere! So, I said no."

This mundane conversation has made no difference. She thinks she has problems, I'm having a bloody root treatment! Then I see the card on the reception desk, a birthday card with a picture of a terrified patient in the chair, with the dentist sitting close by. Next to the patient is the Grim Reaper saying he's come for the patient, but then tells the dentist he can finish the root treatment first. I stifle a silent scream and rush to the toilet.

"Hi Fiona, would you like to come into the surgery?" I see the dentist; he knows his stuff and looks quite sexy in his scrubs. "That's it," I say to myself, "look at him as a sex object!"

THE DENTIST

I look at my day list. Oh fuck! Fiona is coming in last thing for a root treatment and I completely forgot. She will be as nervous as hell and it makes my job really testing. Root treatments are quite routine unless it's a molar tooth at the back, then I usually refer to a specialist who may use a microscope to complete the job.

Dentistry can be like being joined to the patient in an almost intimate fashion. Every movement, every hint of pain I can feel, but in a different way. I feel a sudden tenseness, almost a missed heartbeat, certainly a rapid rise in my pulse. I can see the beads of sweat on the patient, the nervous movements, the hands gripping the chair, and sometimes my leg! I can sense the anticipation when I am injecting the local anaesthetic, the palpable relief when it's finished. When I start the treatment, the tension returns. I can almost feel my blood pressure rising as I start to concentrate. Sudden movement from the patient, a grab for my hand, unnerving! I feel it all.

"Hi Fi, have a seat, I'll talk you through each stage." No response! She's very frightened but I don't think she is going to faint or feel unwell. Now it doesn't matter who the patient is, I will always look to see if there are any signs of distress, and the medical history is always checked and upgraded. I know this patient very, very well, but you can never be sure.

I rub a surface anaesthetic cream on the gum, usually lignocaine based with a flavour — the bubble gum one is very popular and lightens the atmosphere. This will numb the area to be injected. I ask Fi how it feels. "Tingling," she replies. Okay, time for the local anaesthetic (LA), usually an articaine-based one is my favourite. I inject very slowly over the area of the tooth;

this avoids any pain from a sudden increase in pressure from the LA.

I spend the next few minutes talking to the patient. "Where do you fancy going for a holiday?"

Fi looks up at me, grimacing. "Anywhere after this." The nurse smiles in a cryptic fashion.

The next step is to put on a rubber dam. This is a sheet of a rubber like material that fits over the tooth to be treated and isolates the area from saliva and other contamination, whilst at the same time stops instruments from being swallowed or inhaled. Mandatory!

"Okay," I tell Fi. "I'm going to drill a hole in the tooth to locate the nerve canal. The nerve is dead and you've had an anaesthetic, so there will probably be no pain." Shit, I thought, shouldn't have used the word probably. Bad choice.

Tension rises, a doubt in her mind, a mistake. Her hands are gripping the chair tightly and I can see the panic in her eyes. I pick up the high-speed handpiece, touch the tooth, then the whir of the turbine at 250k revolutions per minute. Tentatively, the hole is drilled. Fi relaxes a little, but remains tense. "I have located the root canal and I'm now going to measure the length then clean it out." I look at Fi when saying this with a confident demeanour, followed by a joke to lighten things further. I insert the diagnostic reamer carefully into the canal. No pain. Fi is visibly relieved. Using a digital x-ray that gives an almost immediate image on the monitor, I can see that the reamer is in a good position and with a little basic maths I can determine the true length of the root canal.

The canal is then enlarged with a selection of different sized instruments, and irrigated to clean and disinfect. After the canal is dried, I explain to Fi that I am going to insert the final root filling, and it is possible she would feel a little pressure. Honesty here is the best policy! The final root filling is made up of a pre-measured piece of gutta percha (inert thermoplastic latex from Palaquium tree). I tell Fi this but she is, like my nurse, unimpressed by this information.

"I'm going to put this warm material into the cavity to fill it up," I explain in a most professional voice. For some reason this brings a smile to her face, at last a breakthrough! A final x-ray is taken, and I show her the exact position of the final root filling, accurate and I think very well performed.

"Am I finished now?" Fi asks. No appreciation of my skills!

"Almost, there is just a little hole to fill." She turns towards me and with at last a sparkle in her eyes pleads. "This won't hurt, will it? Because if it does there will be no celebration dinner for us tonight, and you can forget the afters."

"Okay, darling, but I may be a little late. I've got some paperwork to finish off." You know Fi, my wife, is probably my worst patient!

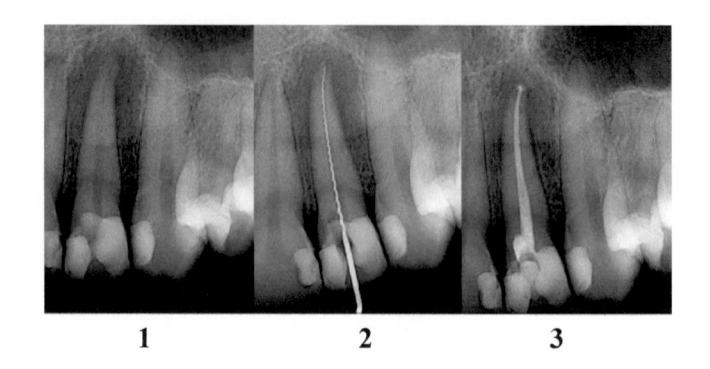

1 BEFORE TREATMENT
2 DIAGNOSTIC REAMER
3 FINAL ROOT TREATMENT

The dark area at the top of the tooth on the first image, before treatment, is an area of infection. The second image shows the diagnostic reamer in position measuring the canal length, whilst the third image shows the final gutta percha root filling completed.

BOOK 3

THE ACCI-DENTAL SLEUTH (IF THE CAP FITS!)

The last patient has just left the surgery and it's a Wednesday. That means a visit to my favourite coffee shop, *Café Noir*, and a piece or two of their special 'cake of the day'. Now I'm very fond of cakes, so Wednesdays are eagerly anticipated. Newspaper in hand I take the short walk to the mecca of sweet treats and sit at my usual window seat so I can watch the world go by for an hour or so.

Mirna, who always serves me, shouts in a loud voice, "Your usual Americano, Doc? And an extra-large piece of lemon drizzle cake with extra drizzle. It will rot your teeth you know!" This is said like a true comedienne, milking the other customers for much mirth and laughter, which was forthcoming. "Thanks," I reply. "Do you know any good dentists?" It's a comment that fell completely on deaf ears, with sundry mutterings about the present costs of NHS treatments. That's it, I think and bury myself in *The Times* sudoku in an effort to revitalise my, by now, jaded brain. I will never be a comedian, and any humorous repost always occurs to me too much later.

Now lemon drizzle cake, if baked properly, combines a light moist sponge infused with a luscious, sharp lemon syrup. It's delicious and the sudden temporary rush of sugar-inspired endorphins sweeps away the traumas of the day.

There's a woman I see every time I'm here. She sits just to my left, and wears the same somewhat weather-beaten coat, and grips a large leather handbag tightly as if it contained her whole life. Her name is Mary. She is slim, early sixties and looks world weary and sad. We are all creatures of habit, and I can tell you exactly what she will order, always English breakfast tea, together with two scones, jam and no butter. Mary sits quietly looking out of the window, with an occasional acknowledgement of some of the other customers. She is always there when I arrive and usually leaves before me.

She pays her bill and leaves. I watch her go and wonder what life had hit her with in her past. Does she have any family? Friends? Or is she going home to an empty house? As she steps out onto the street, she pauses, and an expression of fear fills her face. There is a young man who suddenly confronts her and grabs the handbag. He pulls it, but she resists, yanking it back and hurling it at the face of the thief. He steps back clutching his mouth, then swings a fist at Mary, knocking her to the ground before running off with the bag. In an instant and a blur, it is over. I am out straight away together with some of the other customers, trying to help Mary.

The youth has gone. I catch a glimpse of him on a bike, scuttling off as fast as he can, weaving between the traffic.

We take Mary back inside, give her a cup of her favourite tea, and I examine her to make sure she is free from any obvious injuries. She is distraught. She refuses to go to hospital, claiming she is unhurt, but of more concern is the loss of her handbag. The police are called and a young, very sympathetic policewoman WPC Amil takes all the details, saying the crime will be logged and investigation made. In other words, there is very little chance of getting the handbag back. I do manage a reasonable description of the bike, red, with what seemed to be a crooked rear mudguard. Strangely I think it is a girl's bicycle, with a low bar, but I cannot be sure. "There's been a lot of bike thefts and muggings in the area recently," the WPC says in a resigned tone as if she is fighting an uphill battle. She gives us all her contact details, telling us to call if we have any further concerns.

I tell Mary I will collect my car and take her home. At first, she refuses the offer, but is finally persuaded by all present. I leave her in the café and go out into the street. It is here that something catches my eye on the pavement, a glint in the sunlight, something that should not have been there. I bend down to investigate further. There it is, a gold crown or cap, as it is commonly known, from somebody's mouth. I carefully pick it up, still warm, possibly, but more importantly, covered with saliva and a trace of blood. I carefully wrap it up in a tissue, knowing that it doesn't belong to Mary. She must have knocked it out of the mugger's mouth. Yes! I saw him clutch his face. An important clue!

I don't tell Mary about the crown but am determined to put my forensic skills to work. I take her to her home, not too far away, a modest pretty house and compliment her on her well-kept front garden, bedding plants in full bloom. "The garden is my pride and joy," she says, perked up a little by my observations. "My husband died some years back, and my daughter lives in France now where she works. I don't seem to make friends too easily, so I spend my time in the garden, the local library and the coffee shop. I've seen you there many times but was too shy to talk to you."

"Mary, I hope you don't mind me asking, but what was in the bag? I know you were embarrassed to tell the police."

"You're quite right, I felt so bad about the whole incident. The bag contained all my most precious possessions, photos of my husband Jim, holiday snaps and mementoes such as a pressed flower he gave me when we were married. There was a little money left over from my pension. I was going to get something for dinner on my way home."

I can't leave her as she is. Instead I take her to the local supermarket, and give her some money to pay for food. "I will pay you back," she assures me. "But I don't even know your name."

"Call me Bernard or Doc." I watch her frail figure disappear into her home.

Frail yes, but she has obviously hurt our suspect and I'm sure knocked a crown out. Now, gold crowns are unusual, especially on somebody of his age. They are usually put over a badly damaged tooth and would probably not have been available on the NHS. I examine the crown (cap) in detail with a magnifying glass. Sure enough, still traces of blood stain, but more than that. The yellow gold used looked like a very high quality, definitely made privately. You cannot use pure 24k gold for dental crowns, it's too malleable, so usually an alloy of gold, platinum and palladium is best, with a gold content of at least forty per cent. I need a visit to my technician first for some testing on the crown. Steve is the best I know and I explain to him the situation. It takes him only a few minutes to ascertain the gold content. "It's a high-quality crown Bernard, not only that, I made it." I must have looked a little stunned but Steve goes into the technical details of how he knows this. Suffice to say there is no doubt in his mind. He tells me that he has only made five of these crowns in the last six months, and more, there is a residue of a white powder inside. "This has been cemented in with a temporary cement, as if the dentist wanted to let the tooth settle down before permanently fixing into position.

I leave Steve with a list of dentists that he has made this type of crown for, bless him! I have struck lucky with it, and feel the detective instinct in me taking over. There are three dentists on the list, two in my area and one a little further away, so I will start with the ones nearest to me. Jack Cronshaw qualified at the same hospital in Manchester and he was a little older than me. I make an appointment to see him during his lunch hour and we go through his records to see if we can locate the patient. He had made two gold crowns, both on patients much older than our suspect, so no joy there. I thank Jack who now gives me the nickname 'The Acci-Dental Detective.'

Brian Gosling is not from my area though he qualified in Bristol. He is meticulous in checking the records, photos and x-rays to see if we can locate a possible clue, but no. Again, two cases but much older, and he knows both patients well. "Definitely not our suspect," he says.

I hear from WPC Amil that there has been no progress, and no further sightings of the mugger. She promises to keep me informed and asks me to contact her again if she can help further. Should I tell her about my forensic digging? No, not at this stage I surmise, I am only working on very fragile yet intriguing evidence.

Malcolm Siminof works about twenty miles from my surgery. I contact him, explaining the situation, and that I would like to see him when convenient. To my surprise he says "That's very interesting, can you come straight away after you have finished for the day?"

I feel a slight tingling in anticipation of what Malcolm may have for me, knowing that the chances of tracing our culprit are slim at best. I arrive at his surgery early evening, an old building, immaculately maintained with very up to date equipment. Malcolm lives on the premises with his young family and he is most hospitable, offering me a glass of his finest Mcallan malt whisky, which I reluctantly refuse. "I'm sorry," I explain. "I have to drive back home. Don't let it stop you though," I mutter as I watch him imbibe the amber nectar. "A piece of my wife's finest ginger cake then?" How could I refuse?

"Look at this," Malcolm says. "I have to make a new gold crown for a man aged twenty-two. He's coming to see me the day after tomorrow, apparently. He said he was in an accident and had lost a crown. Does that ring any bells? Not only that, my receptionist reminded me of the last time he was in to fit the original gold crown, about three months ago, a watch went missing from reception. Now we could not categorically say he was responsible, and she did say she was unsure, but hey, some coincidence! He casually decided he wanted to leave his bike in the reception area, concerned it might be stolen if he left it outside. Ironic given what you have told me. That's where we think he may have had access to various personal belongings. "Eureka!" Malcolm suddenly exclaimed, as if the whisky had unlocked a blocked pathway in his brain. "I remember the details now, he was adamant he wanted a gold crown, not a cosmetic one. He joked about being able to trade it in if times got hard. Yes, here it's confirmed in his notes."

I thank Malcolm and leave with an invite for him to come and visit me any time with his young family. "A twenty-three-year-old Glenfiddich will be waiting for you and we can break out a new lemon drizzle cake as well." Malcolm is delighted with the invitation; I can see he is a whisky aficionado. "Keep me informed" are his parting words.

Now the plan could go horribly wrong, we may not have the right person, or he may not turn up for his appointment. Either way arrangements have to be made.

I arrive at Malcolm's surgery early, give him the lost crown, and wait. We have discussed the arrangements in detail, all is set. I sit at a convenient spot away from the reception and waiting room, but in a position where I can see who comes in without being seen myself. His appointment time comes, and goes. A sinking and disappointed feeling comes over me as I move from my hideout towards the reception. Then there is a thud as a bike pushes through the front door. I freeze momentarily as I see the front wheel of a red bike come towards the reception. I compose myself and speedily retreat to my hiding place, and watch. Sure enough, there is the red bike with a low bar, and a crooked back mudguard. "I want to leave it here, it's a rough neighbourhood," he smirks. "Mr. John Carter, isn't it? Please take a seat in the waiting room." The receptionist smiles at him politely, but aware of the possible forthcoming drama. There are two other people in the waiting room as I watch John position himself in a comfortable chair, and pick up a magazine. I wait, then the nurse appears. "Mr. Collier, please follow me into the surgery." I watch him nonchalantly brush past the two other patients, a woman together with a heavily built man who would look more at home in a wrestling arena.

At this signal I hastily put on some scrubs, a face mask and enter the surgery. "Malcolm looks up at me. "Mr Collier, I'm sure you won't mind but I've bought in a colleague to review your case." Our patient looks agitated as he glances round at me, but there is no chance of recognition.

"I had an accident, fell off my bike and I must have lost the gold cap you fitted a few months back. I know you fitted it temporarily, so is it under warranty?" Malcolm is unmoved, but I'm sure I detect a smile behind the mask. I watch as Malcolm picks up the lost crown with practised dexterity, hiding it from Collier's view.

"I'm just going to see if I can fit a temporary crown for you." He slips the crown in place and I watch as it slides on perfectly. "That feels great Doc, just like the lost cap." Malcolm removes his mask and beams." The shoe fits perfectly Cinderella." That is my signal. I leave a bemused looking patient and go straight out to the waiting room, where I signal to WPC Amil and her PC colleague to come into the surgery. As we open the door, we are confronted by the onrushing Collier who has by this time decided that he may be in trouble. As he runs out, he bumps into our PC and seems to bounce off the unmoving constable.

"John Collier, I am arresting you for assault, and theft." WPC Amil twists his arm behind his back whilst reading him his rights.

Malcolm is ecstatic, I don't think he has seen so much excitement in the surgery before. We all take in the scene with a certain amount of satisfaction as Collier is bundled into the back of the unmarked police van, together with important evidence, the bike and the crown, conveniently taken out and placed in a box for future reference.

I am back at my favourite coffee bar; it is a Wednesday. Mary is already there and so I pull up a chair and join her. "How lovely to see you again Mary, how have you been?" She is pleased to see me, telling me her daughter is going to come and see her from France and stay for some time to help out. I can however see that she had not fully recovered from the trauma. What happened next left me close to tears, yet filled with a sense of, well rejuvenation, and a renewed faith in the rare kindness that people are capable of. In walked WPC Amil and the beefy PC, together with Malcolm. I am surprised to say the least, completely lost for words. Poor Mary feared the worst. It seems that they had previously paid a visit to the café, to ascertain when we would both be there.

WPC Amil is carrying a brown paper package, ceremonially placing it on the table. She then almost in a choreographed way, pulls the handbag out, and with a smile that would have lit up a thousand homes, says "I believe this belongs to you Mary. I'm afraid the money has gone, but the photos and that flower and mementos you told me about are still there."

Mary seems to pale before bursting into uncontrolled tears and laughter together, as if something has pulled her out of the darkness in which she had found herself. "I don't know what to say, but thank you, I can't believe you found it."

"Well, we didn't exactly find it, did we Bernard? Suffice to say the culprit will not be around for some time."

With perfect timing, the kitchen door opens and in walks Mirna, carrying a huge lemon drizzle cake and an envelope. Everyone present applauds in what is now a party atmosphere. "I can't eat all that!"

"You won't have to," is the chorus. "We are all going to join in."

Mirna turns to Mary and presents her with the envelope. "Just a little collection we have made for you to help out." Much applause all round from people who were once quiet strangers, but now seem like animated friends. I am lost for words when the owner walks in with a bottle of champagne, pours each a glass and proclaims, "To the Doc, our acci-dental sleuth."

MY BOOK OF LIFE

Life is like a book. It has a beginning, middle and an end. It has many pages, chapters, pauses and full stops. We don't always know what the next page holds. Sometimes we may not want to see it at all. Often life can be a real page turner. We enthusiastically want to keep seeing over, eagerly anticipating what may come next. There is optimism and pessimism, the only difference being that optimists have a better time of things and enjoy their book in a way a pessimist cannot. Life can happen to you when you are planning something else. People plan, God laughs.

There may be an infinite number of stories in your book, where one decision may affect others and have a beneficial or deleterious effect. We are dealt the cards but it is up to us to decide how we play them. The variety of these cards we are born with can affect everything. The colour of our skin, our ethnicity, our socio-economic background, what schools we were allowed to attend and whether it was feasible to have further education. Some of these are now, thankfully, changing for the better — others are not, and may cause serious disruption to life choices.

I was born into a hard-working family, with two older brothers. My father was a teacher, and my mother a seamstress. When I was six or seven, I struggled at school. My mother as astute as ever, realised that it was the school that was at fault due to a lack of teachers. I was moved to a traditional primary school in Crumpsall, Manchester and thrived. Without that decision things may have been very different.

Scholarship passed and then onto the North Manchester Grammar for Boys. A traditional red brick grammar school with a strong headmaster supported by a good teaching staff. I struggled for two years in the lower science stream until I found my feet, and friends such as Gary Simon who I still work with today.

O-levels passed, then another two years in the sixth form, which was part of the school. No need to go to a sixth form college at that time. Gary and I had already decided we were going to apply to Manchester University to study dentistry. Onward and upwards! The A-levels trained me to concentrate, work hard and prepare me for the next step. Physics, Chemistry and Biology all passed by both of us. We were now dental students.

Grants helped with expenses, and would you believe it, we had no tuition fees to pay. If I was confronted with today's costs, I doubt if I could have afforded to complete the course, and be saddled with that amount of debt. Lucky? Absolutely. Look how the cards have now changed for many university courses in this country.

I qualified and walked into a relatively well-paid profession. Then my boss was set to leave the surgery where I had attended as a child for treatment. The option to purchase was offered to me, my first NHS surgery. That was a good card played, but I could have worked elsewhere. I had offers. I could have worked in a hospital. The choice I made was a good chapter in my book. I worked in the NHS for forty years in that surgery. Look at the friends I made, the patients I treated and life lived in a warm working environment, a very good card.

However, nothing was handed to me on a plate. I had to work hard and learn how to run a business — premises to pay for together with wages, materials, taxes and more.

Taking my wife to see a gynaecologist in a building where I eventually took over a private dental practice was another of life's strange coincidences. With the help of excellent staff, I built it up into a successful and well-respected establishment, in the most wonderful place to work, St. John Street, Manchester.

Those two moves to the NHS and private surgeries mapped out my working life. I enjoyed my profession, helped many people and built wonderful working relationships that have endured to this day. I have heard stories that beggar belief, some in this book, and I have still kept in contact with many of these people.

There were many other roads I could have taken, but overall, I consider that I took the best route to fulfil my ambition, my profession, my life.

Humour is a great drug. I will finish with twenty of the best requests that have been made to me. They are all genuine and I hope you will perhaps laugh as I did, when I recalled them.

11. MY TOP TWENTY REQUESTS

PATIENT: Will I grow a third set of teeth; I've got a wedding to go to?
ME: Very unlikely, maybe possible if you come back in a hundred years.

PATIENT: Why does the mint polishing paste you use give me diarrhoea?
ME: That's an anal and banal question to answer.

PATIENT: If I buy two 38e breast implants can you fit them for me?
ME: No, but I would like to see the finished job. (Purely professional interest of course, but this really did happen, what would you have said?)

PATIENT: Can you not make my new crowns too sharp, my boyfriend won't like it?
ME: Erm, I'm not quite sure what you mean.

PATIENT: While I'm here can you have a look at my navel?
ME: It's a bit low for me.

PATIENT: Can I have a gold tooth with a diamond in it on the NHS?
ME: *No.*

PATIENT: I would rather have a baby than a filling!
ME: Please make up your mind, I would have to adjust the chair, but I have tools for both jobs.

PATIENT: Could you check if I'm pregnant please?
ME: I'm sorry but I am only an amateur gynaecologist? (A simple error!)

PATIENT: Is it okay to cement my crown back on with superglue?
ME: No, it contains ethyl cyanoacrylate, breathing in fumes whilst setting is toxic. (I can't believe this!)

PATIENT: I always use VIM to clean my teeth, is it dangerous?
ME: Toilet bleach is meant for toilets, it's concentrated bleach in a powder, does that answer your question? (I'm lost for words!)

POLICE: The prisoner said he had toothache sir; he claims he bought two kilos of cocaine to kill the pain. Would this work?
ME: Excuse me, I just need to call my solicitor!

PATIENT: Can you bring my mobility scooter up the stairs for me?
ME: I'm sorry but I'm not insured to drive it.

PATIENT: I don't like the new dentures you made for me. Can I have a look at some of your second-hand ones please?
ME: Please excuse me I have an urgent call to make.

PATIENT: Can you leave the gap where you extracted the tooth, it just fits a cigarette.
ME: I'm losing the will to go on!

PATIENT: Why are my teeth getting loose, is it the smoking? I've only smoked 30 a day for 40 years.
ME: That's about 27 miles of cigarettes smoked. You are lucky they are only loose.

PATIENT: You have such lovely eyes and voice.
ME: I'm really sorry I can't say the same about your teeth. (Having just extracted her last remaining ones.)

PATIENT: Would you consider marrying my daughter?
ME: I've never met her, and as far as I know bigamy is still an offence in this country. (I wasn't prepared for this at dental school!)

PATIENT: Can you extract a tooth for my cat, you are cheaper than the vet?
ME: *NO.*

PATIENT: Well can you look at my dogs' teeth?
ME: No. (Patience is a virtue never found in men! I need a large Scotch!)

PATIENT ON PHONE: My crown has come off, but my car has broken down and I don't like buses, can you bring your dental chair and everything you need to my house?
ME: To quote my favourite footballer, Vincent Kompany, "That's my lot, I'm done."